Pediatric Bone Sarcomas

Editors

José Cañadell · Mikel San-Julian

Pediatric Bone Sarcomas

Epiphysiolysis Before Excision

Foreword by: Franklin H. Sim

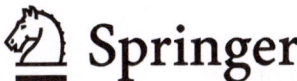

Editors
José Cañadell, MD PhD
Emeritus Professor
Department of Orthopedic Surgery
University of Navarra
Pamplona, Navarra
Spain

Mikel San-Julian, MD PhD
Consultant
Department of Orthopedic Surgery
University of Navarra
Pamplona, Navarra
Spain

ISBN 978-0-85729-517-0 (PB)
ISBN 978-1-84882-129-3 (HB)   e-ISBN 978-1-84882-130-9
DOI 10.1007/978-1-84882-130-9
Springer Dordrecht Heidelberg London New York

British Library Cataloguing in Publication Data
A catalogue record for this book is available from the British Library

Library of Congress Control Number: PCN applied for

Springer is part of Springer Science+Business Media (www.springer.com)

Foreword

Sparing of the growth plate is an early feature of diaphyseal and meta-diaphyseal osteosarcoma. Capitalising on this characteristic, Jose Cañadell has developed an innovative technique to preserve the epiphysis while resecting primary bone malignancies lying adjacent to the growth plate of skeletally immature patients. Using external fixation devices, controlled distraction of the epiphysis from the growth plate permits iatrogenic separation of the epiphysis from the affected region. Subsequent resection is enhanced by a safe distal margin and Cañadell's local control rates attest to the success of the procedure as an oncologically sound technique. The Cañadell technique has been developed through rigorous examination of the behaviour of osteosarcoma, as well as an interrogation of the best modalities for assessing tumour invasion of the growth plate. Combining an innovative treatment philosophy with a sound knowledge of the behaviour of osteosarcoma and basic bone and growth plate biology, as well as an extensive experience with ancillary investigations and adjuvant therapies, Cañadell has developed a robust surgical technique for the management of a challenging tumour in selected patients.

This book is the culmination of Cañadell's endeavours over the last two decades. It traces the steps that he has taken to validate the safety and efficacy of the Cañadell technique as we know it today. Carefully grouped into rationale chapters, this book guides those with a particular interest in musculoskeletal oncology through a technique that they may find valuable when the goal is epiphyseal sparing surgery. The diagrams are clear and the stepwise description of the technique is logical. The selection of histological and anatomic imaging frames has been careful and clearly highlights the important elements underpinning the success of this technique. As a special feature of this book, Cañadell has even included a question and answer section at the end which aims to test whether the educational objectives of his book are being met.

Jose Cañadell's book of techniques is unique and innovative and justifies its place on the shelves of institutions which are focused on advancing the treatment of musculoskeletal tumours.

Rochester, Minessota, USA   Franklin H. Sim

Preface

In the last 30 years, the outcomes achieved with patients affected by malignant bone tumours have improved dramatically. Better knowledge of the disease, improvement of imaging methods, new surgical techniques and particularly the advent of chemotherapy have brought about unanticipated therapeutic successes in this kind of patient.

Thirty years ago, physicians were content if they could preserve the life of these patients; nowadays, however, survival rates continue to improve and the challenge for the orthopaedic surgeon is to preserve the limb and its function and to avoid complications. Thirty years ago, anybody who tried to preserve a joint near a bone tumour would have been considered a fool. Nowadays, this is a realistic goal for everybody who treats these patients.

Since 1984, we have been using in our orthopaedics department a technique which has become increasingly popular among surgeons specialized in bone tumours: physeal distraction (epiphysiolysis) before excision to preserve the joint in metaphyseal bone tumours in children. This little book describes the technique and provides a synopsis of why we use it and how we select which patients to use it with.

Pamplona, Spain

José Cañadell
Mikel San-Julian

Acknowledgments

We like to express our gratitude to everyone who has contributed directly or indirectly to this book, especially to all the team at the Department of Orthopaedic Surgery and Traumatology at the University Clinic of Navarra, whose daily work in the outpatients department, in the operating room and in the laboratory, in conjunction with rigorous research projects, has helped to improve the techniques described and widen their indications.

Our thanks also go to all the specialists from other departments, in particular, the departments of radiology, pediatrics and pathology, who have collaborated with us in this venture, helping us to broaden our perspectives. Whilst this book and the work it outlines is clearly the result of a multidisciplinary effort, there are certain individuals without whom the development of these techniques might never have happened. One of these individuals is Dr. Luis Sierrasesúmaga, Director of the Department of Pediatrics. With his dedication to excellence in research and to the highest standards of treatment and care of children with cancer, he has inspired and supported us throughout our endeavours.

We also thank the nursing personnel: Maite Moyano, Pilar Lacasa, Ana Villanueva, Natividad Iribarren, Carmen Sánchez, Isabel San-Martin and many others, who at all times have been such a dependable and invaluable source of help both to doctors and patients.

Lastly, we like to mention Paz Gúrpide for providing the outline for the book, Javier Gardeta for his presentation of the iconography and David Burdon for his help with translation of the text.

Contents

Contributors

Jesús Dámaso Aquerreta, M.D.
Department of Radiology
University of Navarra
Avda. Pio XII, 36
31008-Pamplona, Spain
e-mail: Jdaquerret@unav.es

Alberto Benito
Department of Radiology
University of Navarra
Avda. Pio XII 36
31080-Pamplona, Spain
e-mail: albenitob@unav.es

José Cañadell
Department of Orthopaedic Surgery
University of Navarra
Avda. Pio XII 36
31080-Pamplona, Spain
e-mail: mmlopez@unav.es

Jose A. Cara, M.D., Ph.D.
Department of Orthopedic Surgery
Marbella Salud, Avda. Ricardo Soriano
36, 1° -, Edificio Maria III
Marbella Malaga 29600, Spain
e-mail: JAC.CARA@terra.es

Maria Dolores Lozano
Department of Patholoy
University of Navarra
Avda. Pio XII 36
31080-Pamplona, Spain
e-mail: mdlozano@unav.es

Francisco Forriol, M.D., Ph.D.
Research Department, FREMAP
Ctra Pozuelo, 61, Majadahonda
Madrid 28220, Spain
e-mail: fforriol@fremap.es

Moira Garraus
Department of Pediatrics
University of Navarra
Avda. Pio XII 36
31008-Pamplona, Spain
e-mail: mgarraus@unav.es

Miguel A. Idoate, M.D., Ph.D.
Department of Pathology
University of Navarra
Avda. Pio XII, 36
31008-Pamplona, Spain
e-mail: maidoate@unav.es

Fernando Lecanda
Oncology Division. Lab 1.02
Center for Applied Medical Research
(CIMA)
University of Navarra
Avda. Pio XII-55
31080-Pamplona, Spain
e-mail: flecanda@unav.es

Mathew J. Most, M.D., Ph.D.
Department of Orthopedic Surgery
Mayo Clinic, 200 First Street SW
Rochester, MN, USA
e-mail: mathewjmost@hotmail.com

Julio de Pablos
Department of Orthopaedic Surgery
Hospital San Juan de Dios
c/ Beloso Alto 3
31006-Pamplona, Spain
e-mail: brupa@ohsjd.es

Ana Patiño-Garcia, M.D., Ph.D.
Laboratory and Department of Pediatrics
University Clinic of Navarra
Irunlarrea SN, Pamplona
Navarra 31080, Spain
e-mail: apatigar@unav.es

Mikel San-Julian, M.D., Ph.D.
Department of Orthopedic Surgery
University of Navarra
Avda. Pio XII, 36
31008-Pamplona, Spain
e-mail: msjulian@unav.es

Luis Sierrasesumaga-Ariznabarreta, M.D., Ph.D.
Department of Pediatrics
University of Navarra
Avda. Pio XII, 36
31008-Pamplona, Spain
e-mail: lsierra@unav.es

Franklin Sim
Department of Orthopaedic Surgery
Mayo Clinic
200 First Street
Rochester 59905, Minessota, USA
e-mail: sim.franklin@mayo.edu

Jesús Vazquez†
Department of Pathology
University of Navarra
Avda Pio XII, 36
31080-Pamplona, Spain

Marta Zalacain
Laboratory and Department of Pediatrics
University Clinic of Navarra
c/Irunlarrea SN
31080-Pamplona, Spain
e-mail: mzalacaind@unav.es

---

†Dr Vazquez died several years ago, but he contributed very much to chapter 5 of this book.

Treatment of Pediatric Bone Sarcomas

1

Luis Sierrasesúmaga-Ariznabarreta and Moira Garraus

Abstract The functional results of surgery are important, but only when the survival of a patient is achieved. The key to success in the overall treatment of malignant bone tumours in children lies in multi-disciplinarity. A good response to chemotherapy together with surgery of quality are both fundamental to treatment success.

Introduction

The optimum treatment of bone tumours affecting children and adolescents requires a multi-disciplinary approach combining surgery, radiotherapy and chemotherapy. Treatment success is based on early diagnosis and on the adequate experience of the medical team; for this reason it is advisable that these cases be treated in centres highly specialized in the management of this pathology.[1]

Malignant bone tumours, with average rates in Europe of the order of 6–7 cases per million, generally represent between 5 and 7% of childhood cancers. The two most frequent types are osteosarcomas and Ewing's tumours. The former constitute a little more than half of bone tumours, the Ewing's tumours over 40%. Chondrosarcomas represent about 2% (rates of the order of 0.1 cases per million). Bone tumours are very infrequent in the very young. Incidence increases with age, up to the 10–14-year-old group, in which a little over 10% of all such tumours occur. Osteosarcomas are very rare before 5 years of age. Until that age, Ewing's tumours are slightly more frequent than are osteosarcomas. In practical terms, the incidence of both types becomes equal in the 5–9-year-old group and, in the 10–14-year-old group the incidence of osteosarcomas overtakes that of the Ewing's tumours. Ewing's sarcomas (ES) are slightly more predominant in males.[2]

Luis Sierrasesúmaga-Ariznabarreta (✉)
Department of Pediatrics, University of Navarra, Pio XII 36, 31008,
Pamplona, Navarra, Spain
e-mail: lsierra@unav.es

J. Cañadell and M. San-Julian (eds.), *Pediatric Bone Sarcomas: Epiphysiolysis Before Excision*,
DOI: 10.1007/978-1-84882-130-9_1, © Springer-Verlag London Limited 2011

Treatment of Osteosarcoma

The bad prognosis initially associated with osteosarcoma patients treated exclusively with local therapy took a turn for the better when chemotherapy was introduced into the treatment schemes in the 1980s. At the time of diagnosis, the best detection methods for metastasis only detect distanced illness in 10–20% of cases.[3] However, without adequate treatment the majority of patients with localized disease will develop metastasis within one year if they only receive local treatment. This means that micrometastases exist at the moment of diagnosis in the majority of patients. With adequate multi-disciplinary treatment, about 70% of patients with localized osteosarcoma can be cured.

Surgery

The objective of surgery is to achieve a "block" resection of the tumour and preserve as much function as possible. Local control can only be achieved with complete resection margins. In accordance with the definitions of Enneking, a complete resection implies the total extirpation of the tumoural tissue (including the biopsy scar) surrounded by an envelope of normal healthy tissue.[4] In the case of a localized osteosarcoma, as opposed to other sarcomas, the possibility of achieving surgical remission is very important for the overall cure.[5] It is for this reason that the primordial objective is to achieve adequate surgical margins at the time of local control surgery. In the past, there has been controversy over the suitability of conservative surgery as opposed to amputation; currently, with modern treatments for conservation of the extremity, local relapse occurs in 4–10% of patients, and there do not seem to be differences between ablation surgery and limb salvage.[5] In the great majority of cases it is going to be possible to carry out surgical techniques that conserve the extremity.[6]

Amputation is currently reserved for those cases in which it not considered possible to resect the primary tumour. During the last few years, the role of conservation surgery has increased markedly. As a result of refinements in neoadjuvant chemotherapy, biomechanical engineering and imaging studies, approximately 90% of patients with osteosarcoma are going to be candidates for conservation surgery.[6]

Chemotherapy

Before the introduction of adjuvant chemotherapy, more than 80% of osteosarcoma patients developed metastatic disease.

The first studies using individual agents began in the 1960s and 1970s and established, on a non-randomized basis, the role of chemotherapy in the management of osteosarcoma.

Responses to individual chemotherapeutic agents such as high doses of methotrexate or doxorubicin were described in 20–40% of patients with metastatic disease.[7]

However, the final demonstration of the importance of systemic treatment in the management of osteosarcoma was not established definitively until the publication of the results of a multi-institutional study, which randomized patients with exclusively surgical treatment versus surgery combined with chemotherapy.[8]

Since then, different combinations of platinum compounds, doxorubicin and high doses of methotrexate have formed the basis of chemotherapy treatments, which cure 50–75% of patients with localized disease.

Lessons from the T-10 Protocols

For over two decades, the treatment of osteosarcoma has followed the basic principles dictated by the T-10 protocol. The T-10 protocol and its variants consist in a chemotherapy regimen with high doses of methotrexate, doxorubicin, cisplatin and a combination of bleomycin, cyclophosphamide and dactinomycin. With the T-10 protocol, the disease-free survival (DFS) at 5 years, as described by its authors, approximates to 70%.[9] In a study undertaken by the European Osteosarcoma Intergroup (EOI), patients were randomized to receive the T-10 protocol or a simpler protocol, with six cycles of a combination of cisplatin and doxorubicin. The final results were equal in the two branches, which suggests that a simple regimen, with cisplatin and doxorubicin, can cure more than half non-metastatic osteosarcoma patients.[10]

One of the greatest contributions of T-10 and its predecessor, T-7, is that the histological response to the neoadjuvant chemotherapy is the most important prognostic factor in patients with localized disease.[11] However, intensification of post-operative or pre-operative therapy with doxorubicin, cisplatin and ifosfamide (IFX) has not improved the results.[12–15]

Ifosfamide or the Ifosfamide–Etoposide Combination in the Treatment of Osteosarcoma

IFX has been incorporated in osteosarcoma treatment regimens. As a result of the first studies, which indicated that IFX as sole agent achieved response rates of 10–60% in patients with refractory disease, some researchers began to use the drug in the rescue of patients with a poor histological response.[16] Originally, IFX doses of 5–8 g/m^2 were used although higher doses (12–18 g/m^2) may be more effective.[17] A study by the Pediatric Oncology Group (POG) in patients with previously untreated metastatic disease demonstrated responses in 27% of cases; the dose used was 12 g/m^2.[17] More recently, IFX has been incorporated as a frontline therapy in the treatment of osteosarcoma under many regimens. However, the final impact of this incorporation is still not clear.[18]

That the joint administration of an alkylating agent with etoposide has a synergistic antitumoural effect has lead to the combined administration of IFX and etoposide in fractionated form over a period of 3–5 days. In patients with refractory osteosarcoma, some of which had previously received IFX, the IFX-etoposide combination gained response rates of 15–48%.[19] Recently, for patients with metastatic osteosarcoma, researchers at the POG incorporated this combination to the basic treatment with cisplatin, doxorubicin and high-dose methotrexate and achieved responses in 62% of patients; the DFS at 2 years was 45%.[17] The combination of IFX with etoposide seems to be more effective than that of IFX alone in patients with metastatic osteosarcoma. These results suggest that future studies should be conducted concerning this combination in the treatment of patients with localized disease. In particular, the use of the IFX-etoposide combination is being used more frequently for the rescue of patients with a poor histological response; however, there is no evidence that this modification to the treatment improves expectations of survival. A joint European-American (EURAMOS) study will try to answer this question with a randomized design. Until the results of this study are complete, it is not advisable to modify post-operative therapy by substituting standard therapy for the IFX-etoposide combination.[20]

The Role of Methotrexate in the Treatment of Osteosarcoma

Methotrexate was one of the first drugs demonstrated to be active in osteosarcoma[21] and has occupied a primordial role in the treatment of osteosarcoma since then. Furthermore, certain evidence suggests that the pharmokinetics of methotrexate can influence the final result, although any such influence is inferior and less clear in the context of more-intensive protocols.[22,23] In any case, the role of methotrexate seems to be limited to administration in high doses (normally 12 g/m^2), given that the administration of lower doses apparently has less impact.[24]

There are no randomized studies investigating the role of methotrexate in the treatment of osteosarcoma. The first EOI study randomized patients to receive six cycles of cisplatin and doxorubicin or four courses of the same combination each preceded by a cycle of high-dose methotrexate.[25] In this study there was an advantage in administering the cisplatin-doxorubicin combination alone: DFS at 5 years was 57% versus 41%. A possible reading of these results is that high doses of methotrexate may not be necessary if other agents are intensified. This interpretation may principally be valid when treatment protocols are followed in countries with fewer resources: where monitorisation of levels is not possible. In Latin America excellent results have been obtained using protocols without methotrexate, protocols that intensify cisplatin, doxorubicin, IFX and etoposide.[26]

Cisplatin and Carboplatin

Cisplatin is one of the most effective agents against osteosarcoma. However, the toxicity of this agent is significant: loss of hearing and renal failure can be permanent in some cases. Both toxicities can be reduced using prolonged infusions. The substitution of carboplatin for cisplatin has been recently evaluated at the St. Jude Children's Research Hospital. In the context of an intense regimen with high doses of methotrexate, IFX and doxorubicin, the use of carboplatin resulted in a DFS at 3 years of 72%, results comparable to treatments using cisplatin, but with much lower toxicity.[18] However, the incorporation of carboplatin in future studies must be evaluated with care, given that recent studies have demonstrated low anti-tumoural effect when it is used alone in patients with metastatic disease.[27] Additionally, even in the context of a multiple regimen, carboplatin is inferior to cisplatin for patients with non-resectable or metastatic osteosarcoma.[28]

Pre-operative Chemotherapy and Intraarterial Chemotherapy

One of the greatest contributions of the T-10 protocol was the recognition that the grade of histological response to pre-operative chemotherapy is the most important prognostic factor in patients with localized disease.[11] This observation has determined most current treatments. Modification of post-operative therapy by intensifying the use of cisplatin, doxorubicin or, more recently, with the incorporation of new agents such as IFX and etoposide have not resulted in significant improvement in the prognosis for patients with poor histological response.[13,14] Exposure of tumoural cells to sub-optimum cytotoxic levels during pre-operative treatment can give rise to the development of chemoresistance and increase the propensity to metastatic dissemination. For this reason, modification of post-operative therapy may no longer be capable of reversing these adverse effects. Following this line of reasoning, the achievement of a fast, early response should be the principal objective. Alternatives to intensification of adjuvant chemotherapy could focus, therefore, on improving the pre-operative treatment. Intensification of pre-operative chemotherapy with cisplatin, doxorubicin and IFX gives rise to a modest increase in the proportion of good responders, but the final impact is minimal.

In the 1980s, Jaffe et al demonstrated that with intraarterial administration it was possible to achieve high concentrations of cisplatin in a tumour without compromising systemic exposure.[29] Following this, various groups included intraarterial administration of cisplatin in their treatment of osteosarcoma. Despite the relevance of this new development, only two groups tried to investigate the matter in a randomized manner. Under the IOR/OS-3 and IOR/OS-5 protocols, researchers at the Instituto Ortopédico Rizzoli randomized patients to receive cisplatin intraarterially or intravenously. In both studies, the pre- and post-operative chemotherapy included doxorubicin and high doses of methotrexate, with the addition of IFX in the second study. In both studies, the proportion of good responders was greater in the group of patients treated with intraarterial cisplatin, but the final results were similar in both groups.[30] Using a similar design, the German study COSS-86 also failed to demonstrate any advantage to intraarterial administration.[31] In a recent study, however, Wilkins et al have described excellent results with this technique.[32]

Treatment of Patients with Metastatic Disease

Approximately 20% of osteosarcoma patients have macroscopic metastatic disease at the time of diagnosis; their prognosis is poor.[32,33] The treatment of these patients must include a very aggressive, multi-disciplinary approach with intensive pre-operative and post-operative chemotherapy and resection of both the primary tumour and metastases.[32,33] Using this approach, contemporary protocols that incorporate IFX or the combination of IFX with etoposide, as well as methotrexate, doxorubicin and cisplatin, have been described to attain rates of DFS at 2 or 5 years of 25–45%[34,35]; a longer follow-up, however, is necessary. Some authors have investigated the use of high-dose chemotherapy and autologous rescue of hematopoietic cells. Whilst this way is feasible, it does not seem to have any advantage over the conventional treatment.[36–38]

For patients with osteosarcoma in relapse, a very aggressive surgical approach is recommended. The survival rate at 5 years after relapse, for patients in whom it is possible to obtain a complete new remission, is approximately 30–40%; it is 0% for patients in whom the disease cannot be resected.[38] The role of chemotherapy seems to be limited to patients with non-resectable disease. The prognostic factors for survival after relapse include the presence of isolated pulmonary metastasis, late relapse (>24 months) and a low number of pulmonary lesions.[38]

Future Treatments

The survival rates for patients with metastatic disease at the time of diagnosis and for those in relapse are very low; less than 30% survive. For this reason it is necessary to develop new strategies, such as new drugs or new combinations, to treat patients with poor prognosis.

The fractionated administration of cyclophosfamide with the inhibitor of topoisomerase, topecan, seems to be a promising combination for the treatment of many pediatric neoplasias. However, in relapsed osteosarcoma patients the rate of response was only 11%, a response far lower than that observed in other neoplasias.[39]

Sequential administration of gemcitabine and docetaxel has been demonstrated to be quite effective in the treatment of sarcomas in relapse. In a study of a group of 35 adult patients with various relapsed sarcomas, the response rate was 43%; in the four patients with refractory osteosarcoma, there were two partial responses and two stable disease states.[40]

Another agent, which has proved to have good activity in vitro against osteosarcoma, is ecteinascidin-743 (ET-743). However, in spite of the promising results of preclinical studies, a phase II study in patients with recurrent osteosarcoma did not demonstrate any activity.[41] It is possible that the role of ET-743 lies in its combination with other chemotherapeutic agents.

The majority of patients who relapse do so with lung metastases. In fact, most patients are considered to have micrometastatic lung disease at the moment of diagnosis. The possibility of controlling this microscopic lung disease on finalizing treatment could give rise to a substantial improvement in survival. In an animal model, the administration of muramyl tripeptide encapsulated in liposomes (L-MTP-PE) activated pulmonary macrophages and brought about the eradication of lung micrometastases.[42] The use of L-MTP-PE is an attractive strategy and requires research. Also, it is possible that one might effect an activation of alveolar macrophages with nebularized GM-CSF. In a phase I study carried out in patients with lung metastasis of various refractory neoplasias, it was possible to nebulize GM-CSF and the toxicity was minimal. The dose tolerated was 250 mcg/dose, twice a day for seven consecutive days every other week. There was a complete response in one patient with an ES and a partial response in a patient with melanoma. Only two patients with osteosarcoma were treated in the study, and in one of them the disease was stabilized for over 11 months.[43] On the basis of these results, the Children's Oncology Group is currently evaluating this treatment in a phase II study involving patients with osteosarcoma with lung metastasis.

Another interesting approach in an animal model is gene transfer of IL-12 by nebularisation using a non-viral vector, such as the cationic DNA transporter polyethylenimine (PEI). Therapy with IL-12 is based on the known anti-tumoural activity of this cytokine. However, the clinical use of IL-12 in a systemic way is limited by its toxicity. Using the technology of PEI:IL-12 transfer in immunosuppressed mice with osteosarcoma lung metastasis, researchers demonstrated an increase in the expression of IL-12 in lung tissue, accompanied by an increase in tissue levels of IL-12. It is important to note that an increased expression of IL-12 in the liver was not observed, which suggests that the systemic effects were minimal. In this animal model, the aerosol therapy brought about a significant decrease in the number of metastatic nodules.[44] Also, it has been demonstrated that IL-12 increases, in vitro, the sensitivity of osteosarcoma to alkylating agents. This occurs through a mechanism involving activation of the Fas pathway. The implication is that IL-12, by aerosol, could have a synergistic effect with IFX. The same technique of PEI transfer has shown anti-tumoural efficiency with transfection of p53.[44]

Aerosolisation technology has extended to the administration of chemotherapeutic agents directly to the lungs. For example, 9-nitrocamptothecin was nebularised into either mice with subcutaneous xenoinserts of a variety of neoplasias or mice with osteosarcoma lung lesions. The results were very satisfactory: good anti-tumoural effect on both the subcutaneous and the lung tumours, which suggests that there is not only a local effect but also a systemic one. Based on these preliminary studies, a phase I study in patients with lung metastasis from refractory neoplasias has recently been completed; phase II studies are being developed.[45]

Finally, administration of high doses of the radiopharmaceutical samarium 153-ethylene diamine tetramethylene phosphate (^{153}Sm-EDTMP) can provide good alleviation of pain with minimal hematological toxicity for patients with local relapse or bone metastasis, and the role of ^{153}Sm-EDTMP as a therapeutic agent could be expanding.[46]

Treatment of Ewing's Sarcoma (ES)

In his initial description of ES as a diffuse endothelioma of the bone, James Ewing pointed out, among other characteristics of this tumour, its elevated susceptibility to radiation therapy.[47] Over the following 50 years, radiotherapy continued to be the predominant way of treating ES, although 80% of patients died after local relapse or metastatic disease during the 2 years after diagnosis.

The current therapeutic approach, which gives cause for much greater optimism in terms of cure rates, seeks to cure the patient while preserving the functionality of the affected body part and to minimize late secondary effects. The approach comprehends a multi-disciplinary focus based on the following concepts:

1. ES has a systemic character at the time of diagnosis. The therapeutic approach requires adequate local control of the macroscopic disease, together with systemic control of micrometastasis.
2. Local control of the macroscopic disease must be multi-disciplinary: combining, according to necessity, surgery, radiotherapy and chemotherapy. The response to neo-adjuvant chemotherapy and the surgical possibilities will determine the doses and fields of radiotherapy. Local control measures must not compromise systemic control.
3. Systemic control of micrometastasis must be carried out through the administration of a protocol of intensive cyclic polychemotherapy comprising agents of the greatest anti-tumoural activity available.
4. Treatment must be adapted to the characteristics of each patient, taking into account the primary localization, the size of the lesion, the staging and therapeutic possibilities according to age. This tailoring is necessary to obtain the maximum therapeutic benefit with the best possible functional result.

Local Control of Disease

Analysis of local control in ES is complicated because of the difficulties involved in the interpretation of the radiological studies usually used in follow-up, after administration of combined treatments. On many occasions, after surgery, radiotherapy and chemotherapy, the signal obtained is not that of a normal bone and is difficult to interpret. Persistence of residual images corresponding to fibrosis, necrosis or both is frequent. In this respect, studies with magnetic resonance after administration of gadolinium are more reliable relative to other imaging techniques.

Consequently, the analysis of results in terms of local control, referred to in the various reported series, which are generally lacking in biopsy/necropsy studies, can under- or overestimate the degree of control. Fernández et al[48] registered a rate of clinical local relapse of 37.5%, which after necroscopic studies, increased to 47.5%. In other studies, even larger differences have been detected: rates of local relapse being 65% while clinical diagnoses scarcely reached 25%.[49]

It is important to note that local control, while an indispensable condition for obtaining a full cure, can, however, accompany a prognosis of death. In the pre-chemotherapy era, rates of local control of 60–70% were reported for series in which the rates of survival were below 20%.[50]

Therapeutic Strategy to Obtain Local Control

Radiotherapy: ES shows great sensitivity to radiation. The local control obtainable with irradiation is directly proportional to the dose administered and to the volume of tissue included in the field. The rate of local control obtainable with radiotherapy is between 50 and 80%. With doses above 40 Gy, high percentages of local control are obtained. With lower doses, even when rapid clinical improvement and disappearance of macroscopic lesions are observed, the incidence of local relapse is very high.[51]

Chemotherapy plus radiotherapy: The addition of chemotherapy protocols to local irradiation have not only meant an advance in the control of systemic disease but have also increased the rates of local disease control. Numerous authors have demonstrated the beneficial effect of this therapeutic association, in comparison with historical series. Consequently, over the last 20 years, this therapeutic focus, which combines high-dose irradiation with systemic chemotherapy, has been considered as optimum in the treatment of ES.[52] The rate of local control that can be expected with the combination of chemotherapy plus radiotherapy is between 75 and 90%.[53-55]

Chemotherapy plus surgery: With the combination of neoadjuvant chemotherapy plus surgery, local control rates similar to those obtained with radiotherapy have been reported.[56] However, it is difficult to compare the two techniques, given that no comparative study of both therapeutic approaches has ever been undertaken. The data of CESS-86 are the closest approximation to a comparative study; differences between both groups were not found (DFS at 5 years was 67% versus 65%).[57] In addition, scrutiny of published works indicates a clear selection of patients. The tendency has been to use surgery for peripheral tumours or for localized tumours of reduced dimensions, which have a better prognosis than central tumours of greater volume.[58] In general there seems to be agreement in the idea of avoiding radiation in patients whose age leads one to predict serious sequelae.

Chemotherapy ± Surgery ± Radiotherapy: Patients who, after induction chemotherapy, demonstrate a high percentage (>30%) of tumour-cell viability in the surgical piece have a bad prognosis. The presence of more than 5% viable tumour is related to low DFS (<5% viable, DFS = 75% versus > 5% viable, DFS = 48%).[59] Similarly, the presence of residual disease in surgical margins or the impossibility of carrying out a complete block resection is associated with a high probability of local relapse.[57,60]

The majority of authors agree in the use of radiotherapy in the following types of patients[61]:

1. Patients for whom there is no surgical option, either initially or after the administration of neoadjuvant chemotherapy.
2. Patients with a bad response to neoadjuvant chemotherapy.
3. Patients in whom no signs of response are observed.
4. Patients in whom there remains residual disease, whether macroscopic or microscopic, in the tumoural bed after surgery.

The figures for local control of disease in patients treated with radiotherapy and chemotherapy are lower for pelvic and proximal locations in comparison to distal locations and for tumours of large initial volume. Various groups have proposed carrying out surgical resection of the zones previously affected by tumour in high-risk patients treated with radiation and chemotherapy. The data obtained in the corresponding series demonstrate a clear advantage in terms of DFS for patients receiving such resection.[62]

Systemic Control of Disease

In the pre-chemotherapy era, survival at 5 years for patients with ES treated with surgery and radiotherapy was less than 10% of cases.[63] As with other childhood solid tumours, phase II studies with sole agents began in the 1960s. All the agents with known activity against solid tumours have been tested, and many of them, as sole agents, demonstrated activity against ES. Out of all of them, cyclophosfamide, IFX, melphalan in high doses and Adriamycin have demonstrated special activity. Other agents such as dactinomycin, BCNU, 5-FU, daunomycin, mitramycin, cisplatin and derivatives of the epipodophyllotoxins have shown different degrees of activity. A combination with surprisingly marked activity, even in patients who are resistant to other drugs, is IFX with etoposide.[64]

The Role of Chemotherapy in Localized Disease

With the anti-tumoural activity of chemotherapy against macroscopic disease proven, in 1964, two of the first studies with complementary chemotherapy were initiated in the St. Jude Children Research Hospital[65] and in National Cancer Institute.[66] Patients were treated with VAC (vincristine, actinomycin D, cyclophosphamide) with or without Adriamycin

(Adr), at doses which we today consider sub-therapeutical. Survival was 33%. In 1973 the first cooperative multi-centre study, denominated IESS-I, began. The study concluded that the addition of Adr to the VAC protocol is effective and better than prophylactic irradiation of the lungs. The VAC + Adr combination obtains a DFS at 5 years of 60%.[52] This study lead on to a second study, the IESS-II, which evaluated the role of intensification of Adr. An increase of 150% of the previous dose improved the DFS at 5 years (73% versus 56%).[67] Studies by other groups with VAC + Adr without intensification achieved very similar results to those obtained in IESS-II.[68] The importance of administering Adr, with VAC, in the highest tolerable doses during the initial stages of treatment is well established.

The development of IFX and the data obtained from phase II studies lead to the idea of substituting cyclophosfamide with IFX. None of the three big studies carried out was able to demonstrate any clear benefit of this substitution. In the control of ES, cyclophosfamide is as effective as IFX in VAC + Adr combinations.[69,70]

Because of the good results obtained with the IFX + VP-16, IESS-III studied the possible benefit of adding this combination to VAC + Adr. A significant increase in the DFS at 5 years was obtained (68% versus 54%).[64]

Currently, for non-metastatic ES chemotherapy treatment, we consider protocols that combine VAC + Adr (in high doses) with IFX + VP-16 as being standard. In a recent study, an adequate combination of this protocol together with surgery and radiotherapy achieved a DFS at 4 years of 82%.[71]

The COG (Children Oncology Group) has proposed carrying out a randomized study to compare the administration of VAC + Adr plus IFX + VP-16 using filgastrim as support, with shorter periods between cycles (14 days versus 21 days), in order to evaluate whether the intensification of doses has an effect on survival. This study is based on the experience of a pilot study by Womer et al,[72] who with this approach obtained a rate of DFS at 30 months of 73%.

Control of Metastatic Disease

The prognosis for patients with metastatic disease is poor. In the majority of series, survival at 3 years is less than 30%.[61,73] Treatment with VACAdr + IFX/E, radiotherapy of foci of macroscopic disease and surgery of resectable lesions makes it possible to reach complete remission in a high percentage of cases. However, the rates of cure do not exceed 20%.[73,74]

The best results with patients with metastatic disease were obtained in a study in the SJCRH by Hayes et al,[75] applying an induction regimen with sequential cyclophosfamide and Adriamycin. The authors report DFS at 47 months of follow-up of 55%. Other authors have not been able to reproduce these results.[76]

According to the data collected by the IESS studies, the addition of IFX and etoposide do not improve the prognosis for metastatic patients.[64] Patients with metastasis exclusively to the lung or pleura or both have a better prognosis: Cure rates reach 30%. These patients must be treated with lung irradiation.[77] For patients with metastasis to bone or bone marrow, the percentage cured is 20–25%. The possibilities of cure for patients with combined forms of metastasis to bone or bone marrow and lung are less than 15%.[73]

The approach to radiotherapy in the treatment of metastatic disease is based on apply-ing the known criteria for localised disease to each of the affected zones. In this way there is an attempt to obtain adequate local control on an area-by-area basis. In most cases it is possible to obtain this control with acceptable morbidity.[78] The problem with carrying out high-dose irradiation of several fields is the limitation this puts on the joint administration of chemotherapy: The radiotherapy can suppose enormous toxicity on the reserve of bone marrow. In patients with lung metastasis, it is necessary to irradiate both pulmonary fields irrespective of whether the nodules disappear as an effect of chemotherapy.[77] The doses recommended are between 12 and 15 Gy and must be modulated according to the existing pulmonary function.

Analysis of the results obtained with high-dose chemotherapy with or without fullbody irradiation and support with haematopoietic stem cells from bone marrow or peripheral blood is not conclusive. Although some authors, usually with small series of patients, sug-gest an improvement in survival in high-risk situations,[79-81] studies with larger series have not confirmed this therapeutic benefit.[82,83]

Relapse or Progression of Disease

Despite the extensive therapeutic efforts carried in the treatment of ES, between 30 and 40% of patients relapse. The prognosis for patients who present relapse or disease progres-sion before having attained complete remission is very poor. This prognosis is especially bad if progression occurs during chemotherapy treatment.[84,85] Patients with late relapse, that is, over 24 months after diagnosis, have a better prognosis than those with early relapse (34.9% ± 8.5% versus 5% ± 2.8%).

Multiple relapses, local and systemic, are associated with lower rates of survival at 5 years (12.5% ± 8.3%) than local relapse alone (21.7% ± 7.8%) or relapse at a distance alone (17.6% ± 6.1%).[84] For patients with local relapse, radical rescue surgery is the treat-ment, which offers the highest probability of survival at 5 years (31.4% ± 11.6%); alterna-tive treatments are less effective (9.1% ± 6.1%). Lung irradiation significantly improves survival of patients with progression exclusively in this area (DFS at 5 years of 30.3% ± 12.5% versus 16.7 ± 10.8%).[84]

The approach to treatment aimed at the re-induction of remission is very variable and depends on the situation of the patient, on the localisation of the relapse, and on treatment previously received. In patients who have not received it previously, the combination of IFX with etoposide is active: response rates of 80%, the majority partial and 12% com-plete, have been described.[86] In addition, there are reports of responses to the combination of cyclophosfamide with topotecan, with rates of 35% (RC + RP).[87]

When confronted with a well-localized lesion, surgical rescue complemented with local irradiation of the tumoural space can be considered if the relevant tissue has not already been treated.[84]

Treatments with high-dose chemotherapy and rescue with hematopoietic stem cells have been applied by multiple workgroups. The results are better if the procedure is carried out with the patient in complete remission, or at least in a phase in which the disease is contained. Differences between autologous and alogenic transplant have not been found.

The rate of survival at 5 years with these treatments is 24% ± 7%.[88] Before carrying out an autologous transplant it is necessary to make sure, by means of RT-PCR, that the insert is not a carrier of malignant cells. With regard to the regimen of chemotherapy to be used for the induction of remission, the European Bone Marrow Transplant Registry has suggested that the inclusion of busulfan improves results.[89]

New Biological Approaches

In a search for new treatments, Mitsiades et al,[90] after demonstrating that TRAIL (TNF-related apoptosis-inducing ligand) bound with the DR4 and DR5 cellular death receptors, found an elevated expression of DR4/DR5 in samples of ES and high sensitivity to TRAIL in cell cultures. Given the low toxicity of TRAIL, these authors suggested its use as an anti-tumoural agent.

Zhou et al[91] maintain the theory that over-expression of the HER2/neu oncogene is associated with tumourigenicity and resistance to drugs in many human tumours. In three cell lines of human ES it has been demonstrated that the expression of high levels of the protein HER2/neu can be transduced with the E1A gene using an adenoviral vector. In this way it is possible to deregulate the over-expression of the HER2/neu gene, increase cytostasis and reinforce expression of topoisomerase II-alpha. Apoptosis is increased in the tumoural cell lines and there is improved sensitivity to etoposide and Adriamycin.

The receptor for stem-cell factor/KIT could represent a new target for ES treatments of the biological type. Of Ewing's tumours, 44.5% express KIT. Treatments with the tyrosine kinase inhibitor of KIT, imatinib, induce a slowing down in the phosphorylation of KIT and a dose-response inhibition of cellular proliferation. Imatinib administered alone does not induce an important increase of cellular apoptosis, but it has been demonstrated that it increases the toxic action of cytostatics such as vincristine and Adriamycin. Through this mechanism, imatinib could play an important role in the treatment of ES.[92]

References

1. Bielack SS, Machatschek J-N, Flege S, Jürgens H. Delaying surgery with chemotherapy for osteosarcoma of the extremities. *Expert Opin Pharmacother*. 2004;5:1243–1256.
2. Peris-Bonet R, Giner Ripoll B, García Cano A. *Registro Nacional de Tumores Infantiles (RNTI-SEOP). Estadísticas Básicas 4. 1980–2001. Supervivencia 1980–1997*. Valencia: Universitat de València, 2003 (CD-ROM).
3. Jaffe N, Frei E, Traggis D, Bishop Y. Adjuvant methotrexate and citrovorum-factor treatment of osteogenic sarcoma. *N Engl J Med*. 1974;291:994–997.
4. Enneking WF, Spanier SS, Goodman MA. A system for the surgical staging of musculoskeletal sarcoma. *Clin Orthop*. 1980;153:106–120.
5. Bielack SS, Kempf-Bielack B, Delling G, et al. Prognostic factors in high-grade osteosarcoma of the extremities or trunk: an analysis of 1,702 patients treated on neoadjuvant Cooperative Osteosarcoma Study Group Protocols. *J Clin Oncol*. 2002;20:776–790.
6. Bacci G, Ferrari S, Longhi A, et al. Pattern of relapse in patients with osteosarcoma of the extremities treated with neoadjuvant chemotherapy. *Eur J Cancer*. 2001;37:32–38.

7. Cortes EP, Holland JF, Wang JJ, et al. Amputation and Adriamycin in primary osteosarcoma. *N Engl J Med.* 1974;291:998–1000.

8. Link MP, Goorin AM, Miser AW, et al. The effect of adjuvant chemotherapy on relapse-free survival in patients with osteosarcoma of the extremity. *N Engl J Med.* 1986;314:1600–1606.

9. Rosen G, Caparros B, Huvos AG, et al. Preoperative chemotherapy for osteogenic sarcoma: selection of postoperative adjuvant chemotherapy based on the response of the primary tumor to preoperative chemotherapy. *Cancer.* 1982;49:1221–1230.

10. Bramwell VHC, Burgers M, Sneath R, et al. A comparison of two short intensive adjuvant chemotherapy regimens in operable osteosarcoma of limbs in children and young adults: the first study of the European Osteosarcoma Intergroup. *J Clin Oncol.* 1992;10:1579–1591.

11. Meyers PA, Heller G, Healey J, et al. Chemotherapy for nonmetastatic osteogenic sarcoma: the Memorial Sloan-Kettering Experience. *J Clin Oncol.* 1992;10:5–15.

12. Ferrari S, Bacci G, Picci P, et al. Long-term follow-up and post-relapse survival in patients with non-metastatic osteosarcoma of the extremity treated with neoadjuvant chemotherapy. *Ann Oncol.* 1997;8:765–771.

13. Ferrari S, Bacci G, Picci P, et al. Long-term follow-up and post-relapse survival in patients with non-metastatic osteosarcoma of the extremity treated with neoadjuvant chemotherapy. *Ann Oncol.* 1997;8:765–771.

14. Provisor AJ, Ettinger LJ, Nachman JB, et al. Treatment of nonmetastatic osteosarcoma of the extremity with preoperative and postoperative chemotherapy: a report from the Children's Cancer Group. *J Clin Oncol.* 1997;15:76–84.

15. Winkler K, Beron G, Delling G, et al. Neoadjuvant chemotherapy of osteosarcoma: results of a randomized cooperative trial (COSS-82) with salvage chemotherapy based on histological tumor response. *J Clin Oncol.* 1988;6:329–337.

16. Harris MB, Cantor AB, Goorin AM, et al. Treatment of osteosarcoma with ifosfamide: comparison of response in pediatric patients with recurrent disease versus patients previously untreated: a Pediatric Oncology Group study. *Med Pediatr Oncol.* 1995;24:87–92.

17. Goorin AM, Harris MB, Bernstein M, et al. Phase II/III trial of etoposide and high-dose ifosfamide in newly diagnosed metastatic osteosarcoma: a Pediatric Oncology Group trial. *J Clin Oncol.* 2002;20:426–433.

18. Meyer WH, Pratt CB, Poquette CA, et al. Carboplatin/ifosfamide window therapy for osteosarcoma: Results of the St Jude Children's Research Hospital OS-91 trial. *J Clin Oncol.* 2001;19:171–182.

19. Gentet J-C, Brunat-Mentigny M, Demaille MC, et al. Ifosfamide and etoposide in childhood osteosarcoma. A phase II study of the French Society of Paediatric Oncology. *Eur J Cancer.* 1997;33:232–237.

20. Smeland S, Müller C, Alvegård TA, et al. Scandinavian Sarcoma Group Osteosarcoma Study SSG VIII: prognostic factors for outcome and the role of replacement salvage chemotherapy for poor histological responders. *Eur J Cancer.* 2003;39:488–494.

21. Jaffe N, Frei E, Traggis D, Bishop Y. Adjuvant methotrexate and citrovorum-factor treatment of osteogenic sarcoma. *N Engl J Med.* 1974;291:994–997.

22. Graf N, Winkler K, Betlemovic M, Fuchs N, Bode U. Methotrexate pharmacokinetics and prognosis in osteosarcoma. *J Clin Oncol.* 1994;12:1443–1451.

23. Crews KR, Liu T, Rodriguez-Galindo C, et al. High-dose methotrexate pharmacokinetics and outcome of children and young adults with osteosarcoma. *Cancer.* 2004;100:1723–1733.

24. Bacci G, Picci P, Ruggieri P, et al. Primary chemotherapy and delayed surgery (neoadjuvant chemotherapy) for osteosarcoma of the extremities. *Cancer.* 1990;65:2539–2553.

25. Bramwell VHC, Burgers M, Sneath R, et al. A comparison of two short intensive adjuvant chemotherapy regimens in operable osteosarcoma of limbs in children and young adults: the first study of the European Osteosarcoma Intergroup. *J Clin Oncol.* 1992;10:1579–1591.

26. Petrilli AS, Oliveira DT, Ginani VC, et al. Use of amifostine in the therapy of osteosarcoma in children and adolescents. *J Pediatr Hematol Oncol*. 2002;24:188–191.

27. Ferguson WS, Harris MB, Goorin AM, et al. Presurgical window of carboplatin and surgery and multidrug chemotherapy for the treatment of newly diagnosed metastatic or unresectable osteosarcoma: Pediatric Oncology Group trial. *J Pediatr Hematol Oncol*. 2001;23:340–348.

28. Daw NC, Rodriguez-Galindo C, Billups CA, et al. Metastatic osteosarcoma: results of two consecutive therapeutic trials at St. Jude Children's Research Hospital. *Proc Annu Meet Am Soc Clin Oncol*. 2002;21.

29. Jaffe N, Knapp J, Chuang VP, et al. Osteosarcoma: intra-arterial treatment of the primary tumor with cis-diammine-dichloroplatinum II (CDP). *Cancer*. 1983;51:402–407.

30. Bacci G, Ferrari S, Tienghi A, et al. A comparison of methods of loco-regional chemotherapy combined with systemic chemotherapy as neo-adjuvant treatment of osteosarcoma of the extremity. *Eur J Surg Oncol*. 2001;27:98–104.

31. Winkler K, Bielak S, Delling G, et al. Effect of intraarterial versus intravenous cisplatin in addition to systemic doxorubicin, high-dose methotrexate, and ifosfamide on histologic tumor response in osteosarcoma (study COSS-86). *Cancer*. 1990;66:1703–1710.

32. Wilkins RM, Cullen JW, Odom L, et al. Superior survival in treatment of primary nonmetastatic pediatric osteosarcoma of the extremity. *Ann Surg Oncol*. 2003;10:498–507.

33. Kager L, Zoubek A, Pötschger U, et al. Primary metastatic osteosarcoma: presentation and outcome of patients treated on neoadjuvant Cooperative Osteosarcoma Study Group protocols. *J Clin Oncol*. 2003;21:2011–2018.

34. Bacci G, Briccoli A, Rocca M, et al. Neoadjuvant chemotherapy for osteosarcoma of the extremities with metastases at presentation: recent experience at the Rizzoli Institute in 57 patients treated with cisplatin, doxorubicin, and a high dose of methotrexate and ifosfamide. *Ann Oncol*. 2003;14:1126–1134.

35. Bacci G, Briccoli A, Ferrari S, et al. Neoadjuvant chemotherapy for osteosarcoma of the extremity: long-term results of the Rizzoli's 4th protocol. *Eur J Cancer*. 2001;37:2030–2039.

36. Fagioli F, Aglietta M, Tienghi A, et al. High-dose chemotherapy in the treatment of relapsed osteosarcoma: an Italian Sarcoma Group Study. *J Clin Oncol*. 2002;20:2150–2156.

37. Kasper B, Lehnert T, Bernd L, et al. High-dose chemotherapy with autologous peripheral blood stem cell transplantation for bone and soft-tissue sarcomas. *Bone Marrow Transplant*. 2004;34:37–41.

38. Ferrari S, Briccoli A, Mercuri M, et al. Postrelapse survival in osteosarcoma of the extremities: prognostic factors for long-term survival. *J Clin Oncol*. 2003;21:710–715.

39. Saylors RL, Stine KC, Sullivan J, et al. Cyclophosphamide plus topotecan in children with recurrent or refractory solid tumors: a pediatric oncology group (POG) phase II study. *J Clin Oncol*. 2001;19:3463–3469.

40. Leu KM, Ostruszka LJ, Shewach D, et al. Laboratory and clinical evidence of synergistic cytotoxicity of sequential treatment with gemcitabine followed by docetaxel in the treatment of sarcoma. *J Clin Oncol*. 2004;22:1706–1712.

41. Laverdiere C, Kolb EA, Supko JG, et al. Phase II study of ecteinascidin 743 in heavily pretreated patients with recurrent osteosarcoma. *Cancer*. 2003;98:832–840.

42. Kleinerman ES. Biologic therapy for osteosarcoma using liposome-encapsulated muramyl tripeptide. *Hematol Oncol Clin North Am*. 1995;9:927–938.

43. Anderson PM, Markivic SN, Sloan JA, et al. Aerosol granulocyte macrophage-colony stimulating factor: a low toxicity, lung-specific biological therapy in patients with lung metastases. *Clin Cancer Res*. 1999;2316–2323.

44. Densmore CL, Kleinerman ES, Gautam A, et al. Growth suppression of established human osteosarcoma lung metastases in mice by aerosol gene therapy with PEI-*p53* complexes. *Cancer Gene Ther*. 2001;8:619–627.

45. Verschraegen CF, Gilbert BE, Loyer E, et al. Clinical evaluation of the delivery and safety of aerosolized liposomal 9-nitro-20(S)-camptothecin in patients with advanced pulmonary mallignancies. *Clin Cancer Res*. 2004;10:2319–2326.

46. Bacci G, Ferrari S, Bertoni F, et al. Long-term outcome for patients with nonmetastatic osteosarcoma of the extremity treated at the Istituto Ortopedico Rizzoli according to the Istituto Ortopedico Rizzoli/Osteosarcoma-2 protocol: an updated report. *J Clin Oncol*. 2000;18:4016–4027.

47. Ewing J. Diffuse endotelioma of bone. *Proc NY Pathol Soc*. 1921;21:17–24.

48. Fernández CH, Lindberg RD, Sutow WW, Samuels ML. Localized Ewing's sarcoma - treatment and results. *Cancer*. 1974;34:143–148.

49. Tepper J, Glaubiger D, Lichter A, et al. Local control of Ewing's sarcoma of bone with radiotherapy and combination chemotherapy. *Cancer*. 1980;46:1969–1973.

50. Dahlin DC, Coventy MD, Scanlon PW. Ewing's sarcoma: a critical analysis of 165 cases. *J Bone Joint Surg Am*. 1962;43:185–192.

51. Suit HD. Role of therapeutic radiology in cancer of bone. *Cancer*. 1975;35:930–935.

52. Nesbit ME Jr, Gehan EA, Burget EO, et al. Multimodal therapy for the managament of primary, nonmetastatic Ewing's sarcoma of bone: a long-term follow up of the First Intergroup study. *J Clin Oncol*. 1990;8:1664–1674.

53. Shuck A, Hofmann J, Rube C, et al. Radiotherapy in Ewing's sarcoma and PNET of the chest wall: results of the trials CESS 81, CESS 86 and EICESS 92. *Int J Radiat Oncol Biol Phys*. 1998;42:1001–1006.

54. Shankar AG, Pinkerton CR, Atra A, et al. Local therapy and other factors influencing site of relapse in patients with with localised Ewing's sarcoma. *Eur J Cancer*. 1999;35:1698–1704.

55. Rosito P, Mancini AF, Rondelli R, et al. Italian Cooperative Study for the treatment of children and young adults with localized Ewing sarcoma of bone: a preliminary report of 6 years of experience. *Cancer*. 1999;86:421–428.

56. Yaw KM. Pediatric bone tumors. *Semin Surg Oncol*. 1999;16:173–183.

57. Dunst J, Jurgens H, Sauer R, et al. Radiation therapy in Ewing's sarcoma: an update of the CESS 86 trial. *Int J Radiat Oncol Biol Phys*. 1995;32:919–930.

58. Paulussen M, Ahrens S, Dunst J, et al. Localized Ewing tumor of bone: final results of the cooperative Ewing's Sarcoma Study CESS 86. *J Clin Oncol*. 2001;19:1818–1829.

59. Oberlin O, Deley MC, Bui BN, et al. French Society of Paediatric Oncology: Prognostic factors in localized Ewing's tumors and peripheral neuroectodermal tumors: the third study of the French Society of Paediatric Oncology (EW88 study). *Br J Cancer*. 2001;85:1646–1654.

60. Scully SP, Temple HT, O'Keefe RJ, et al. Role of surgical resection in pelvic Ewing's sarcoma. *J Clin Oncol*. 1995;13:2336–2341.

61. Ginsberg JP, Woo SY, Johnson ME, Hicks MJ, Horowitz ME. Ewing's sarcoma family of tumors: Ewing's sarcoma of bone and soft tissue and peripheral primitive neuroectodermal tumors. In: Pizzo P, Poplack D, eds. Principles and Practice of Pediatric Oncology, 4th ed. Philadelphia: Lippincott Williams & Wilkins; 2002:973–1016.

62. Givens SS, Woo SY, Huang LY, et al. Non metastatic Ewing's sarcoma: twenty years of experience suggest that surgery is a prime factor for successful multimodality therapy. *Int J Radiat Oncol Biol Phys*. 1999;14:1039–1043.

63. Wang CC, Schultz MD. Ewing's sarcoma. *N Engl J Med* 1953;248:371–376.

64. Grier HE, Krailo MD, Tarbell NJ, et al. Addition of ifosfamide and etoposide to standard chemotherapy for Ewing's sarcoma and primitive neuroectodermal tumor of bone. *N Engl J Med*. 2003;348:694–701.

65. Hustu HO, Pinkel D, Pratt CB. Treatment of clinically localized Ewing's sarcoma with radiotherapy and chemotherapy. *Cancer*. 1972;30:1522–1527.

66. Tepper J, Glaubiger D, Lichter A, et al. Local control of Ewing's sarcoma of bone with radiotherapy and combination chemotherapy. *Cancer*. 1980;46:1969–1973.

67. Burgert EO, Nesbit ME, Garnsey LA, et al. Multimodal therapy for the management of nonpelvic, localized Ewing's sarcoma of bone: intergroup study IESS-II. *J Clin Oncol.* 1990;8:1514–1524.

68. Hayes FA, Thompson EI, Parvey L, et al. Metastatic Ewing's sarcoma: remission induction and survival. *J Clin Oncol.* 1987;5:1199–1204.

69. Jurgens H, Ahrens S, Frohlich B, et al. European Intergroup Cooperative Ewing's Sarcoma Study (EICESS-92): first results. *Proc Am Soc Clin Oncol.* 2000;19:581a.

70. Oberlin O, Habrand JL, Zucker JM, et al. No benefit of ifosfamide in Ewing's sarcoma: a non randomized study of FSPO. *J Clin Oncol.* 1992;10:1407–1412.

71. Kolb EA, Kushner BH, Gorlick R, et al. Long-term event-free survival after intensive chemotherapy for Ewing's family of tumors in children and young adults. *J Clin Oncol.* 2003;21:3423–3430.

72. Womer RB, Daller RT, Fenton JG, et al. Granulocyte colony stimulating factor permits dose intensification by interval compression in the treatment of Ewing's sarcomas and soft tissue sarcomas in children. *Eur J Cancer.* 2000;36:87–94.

73. Paulussen M, Ahrens S, Craft AW, et al. Ewing's tumors with primary lung metastases: survival analysis of 114 (European Intergroup Cooperative Ewing's Sarcoma Studies) patients. *J Clin Oncol.* 1998;16:3044–3052.

74. Pinkerton CR, Bataillard A, Guillo S, et al. Treatment strategies for metastatic Ewing's sarcoma. *Eur J Cancer.* 2001;37:1338–1344.

75. Hayes FA, Thompson EI, Parvey L, et al. Metastatic Ewing's sarcoma: remission induction and survival. *J Clin Oncol.* 1987;5:1199–1204.

76. Michon J, Oberlin O, Demeocq F, et al. Poor results in metastatic Ewing's sarcoma treated according to the scheme of the St. Jude 1978–1985 study: a study of the FSPO. SIOP XXV Meeting. *Med Pediatr Oncol.* 1993;21:572.

77. Paulussen M, Ahrens S, Burdach S, et al. Primary metastatic (stage IV) Ewing tumor: survival analysis of 171 patients from the EICESS studies. European Intergroup Cooperative Ewing Sarcoma Studies. *Ann Oncol.* 1998;9:275–281.

78. Donaldson SS, Torrey M, Link MP, et al; for Pediatric Oncology Group. A multidisciplinary study investigating radiotherapy in Ewing's sarcoma: end results of POG #8346. *Int J Radiat Oncol Biol Phys* 1998;42:125–135.

79. Atra A, Whelan JS, Calvagna V, et al. High-dose busulfan/melphalan with autologous stem cell rescue in Ewing's sarcoma. *Bone Marrow Transplant.* 1997;20:843–846.

80. Madero L, Muñoz A, Sánchez de Toledo J, et al. Megatherapy in children with high-risk Ewing's sarcoma in first complete remission. *Bone Marrow Transplant.* 1998;21:795–799.

81. Perentesis J, Katsanis E, DeFor T, et al. Autologous stem cell transplantation for high risk pediatric solid tumors. *Bone Marrow Transplant.* 1999;24:609–615.

82. Horowitz ME, Kinsella TJ, Wexler LH, et al. Total-body irradiation and autologous bone marrow transplant in the treatment of high-risk Ewing's sarcoma and rhabdomyosarcoma. *J Clin Oncol.* 1993;11:1911–1918.

83. Meyers PA, Krailo MD, Ladanyi M, et al. High-dose melphalan, etoposide, totalbody irradiation, and autologous stem-cell reconstitution as consolidation therapy for high-risk Ewing's sarcoma does not improve prognosis. *J Clin Oncol.* 2001;19:2812–2820.

84. Rodriguez-Galindo C, Billups CA, Kun LE, et al. Survival after recurrence of Ewing tumors: the St Jude Children's Research Hospital experience, 1979–1999. *Cancer.* 2002;94:561–569.

85. Shankar AG, Ashley S, Craft AW, et al. Outcome after relapse in an unselected cohort of children and adolescents with Ewing sarcoma. *Med Pediatr Oncol.* 2003;40:141–147.

86. Miser JS, Kinsella TJ, Triche TJ, et al. Ifosfamide with mesna uroprotection and etoposide: an effective regimen in the treatment of recurrent sarcomas and other tumors of children and young adults. *J Clin Oncol.* 1987;5:1191–1198.

87. Saylors RL III, Stine KC, Sullivan J, et al. Cyclophosphamide plus topotecan in children with recurrent or refractory solid tumors: a Pediatric Oncology Group phase II study. *J Clin Oncol.* 2001;19:3463–3469.

88. Burdach S, van Kaick B, Laws HJ, et al. Allogeneic and autologous stem-cell transplantation in advanced Ewing tumors. An update after long-term follow-up from two centers of the European Intergroup study EICESS. Stem-Cell Transplant Programs at Düsseldorf University Medical Center, Germany and St. Anna Kinderspital, Vienna, Austria. *Ann Oncol.* 2000;11(11): 1451–1462.
89. Diaz MA, Vicent MG, Madero L. High-dose busulfan/melphalan as conditioning for autologous PBPC transplantation in pediatric patients with solid tumors. *Bone Marrow Transplant.* 1999;11:1157–1159.
90. Mitsiades N, Poulaki V, Mitsiades C, et al. Ewing's sarcoma family tumors are sensitive to tumor necrosis factor-related apoptosis-inducing ligand and express death receptor 4 and death receptor 5. *Cancer Res.* 2001;61:2704–2712.
91. Zhou Z, Jia SF, Hung MC, et al. E1A sensitizes HER2/neu-overexpressing Ewing's sarcoma cells to topoisomerase II-targeting anticancer drugs. *Cancer Res.* 2001;61:3394–3398.
92. Gonzalez I, Andreu EJ, Panizo A, et al. Imatinib inhibits proliferation of Ewing tumor cells mediated by the stem cell factor/KIT receptor pathway, and sensitizes cells to vincristine and doxorubicin-induced apoptosis. *Clin Cancer Res.* 2004;10:751–761.

Molecular Biology of Pediatric Bone Sarcomas

Ana Patiño-Garcia, Marta Zalacain-Diez, and Fernando Lecanda

Abstract Genetic studies can help in diagnosis, prognosis and treatment of pediatric bone sarcoma patients. On the basis of recent discoveries, new drugs (targeted therapies) to help cure these patients are being developed.

Osteosarcoma

Genetic Alterations

The molecular pathways involved in osteosarcoma development are complex and have not been fully explored, and their implication in the development and prognosis of this childhood tumour are not well understood. Even though certain clinical markers are clearly associated with prognosis, their value is limited by the fact that they become evident in stages of the tumoural process which are advanced: development of metastases, relapse and response to neo-adjuvant chemotherapy. It is becoming imperative to determine early molecular markers that allow for a more rationale use of chemotherapy, for the development of new effective treatments and for the stratification of patients according to risk.[1]

In this chapter, we will give a concise description of the pathways most frequently associated with osteosarcoma development and pathways that have been proved to have a prognostic value.

Angiogenesis

The vascular endothelial growth factor (VEGF) stimulates microvascular growth and has an outstanding role in the development of certain tumours (breast, colon, etc.) by increasing the supply of nutrients and blood to them. The use of anti-angiogenic agents

Ana Patiño-Garcia (✉)
Laboratory and Department of Pediatrics, University Clinic of Navarra, Irunlarrea SN, Pamplona, Navarra 31080, Spain
e-mail: apatigar@unav.es

J. Cañadell and M. San-Julian (eds.), *Pediatric Bone Sarcomas: Epiphysiolysis Before Excision*, DOI: 10.1007/978-1-84882-130-9_2, © Springer-Verlag London Limited 2011

(inhibitors of the VEGF pathway) is controversial in the case of osteosarcoma, and reports show contradictory results.[2,3] Therefore, the utility of this and other related molecules [pigment epithelium derived factor (PEDF)] as therapeutic targets in osteosarcoma and their synergic effect with chemotherapy has yet to be determined, with studies already in progress.[4]

Matrix Metalloproteinases

Matrix metalloproteinases (MMPs) are enzymes that are physiologically involved in tissue remodelling and angiogenesis. Excessive production of MMPs, whether as a result of increased transcription of coding genes or of a lack of inhibitors, is important in the process of invasion and metastasis. MMP9, a member of this family, seems to have a prominent role in bone remodelling diseases like osteosarcoma, and several publications have shown that MMP9 overexpression is a poor prognostic factor in osteosarcoma (with an increase in metastatic potential and reduced 5-year overall survival).[5,6] MMP9 can be repressed by a variety of molecules, a fact that makes it an interesting target for attempts to decrease the invasive potential of tumour cells. Indeed, this effect has been demonstrated in animal models and cultured cells.

P Glycoprotein

P glycoprotein (P-gp), which is codified by the multidrug resistance 1 (MDR1) gene, is a membrane molecule involved in drug transport. For more than a decade P-gp overexpression has been known to be a poor prognostic factor in osteosarcoma.[7] There are various reasons for this, one of them being that it is the mechanism by which osteosarcoma cells become resistant to doxorubicin, a prime cytostatic drug in the standard chemotherapy for this pediatric tumour.[8]

Some authors have identified a link between P-gp and p53 overexpression. The p53 molecular pathway is another pathway frequently altered in this type of tumour. According to this model, those patients whose tumours have an altered coexpression of P-gp and p53 would have significantly reduced survival and a more unfavourable Enneking stage.[9]

Cell Cycle Control

Alteration of the different components of the pathway of cell cycle control, particularly those of the p53 and retinoblastoma (RB1) pathways, seems to be the hallmark of the carcinogenic process underlying pediatric osteosarcoma: an alteration in the p53 pathway, the RB1 pathway or both has been detected in most tumours.[10]

The p53 Pathway

Alterations that lead to inactivation of the p53 tumour suppression gene are frequently found in sporadic human tumours. The result is a loss of control of the cell cycle and the DNA repair mechanisms (Fig. 2.1). Although there is considerable published evidence suggesting that the p53 protein has a role in the development of both sporadic osteosarcomas and those associated with the Li–Fraumeni syndrome,[11] the prognostic value of such alterations has not been definitely established.[12,13]

The RB1 Pathway

The cell cycle control pathway that includes the retinoblastoma gene, RB1, is frequently altered in human tumours, especially in osteosarcomas[14] (Fig. 2.1). As described later, the loss of genetic material affecting the long arm of chromosome 13 (13q14) is a frequent genetic event in primary osteosarcomas, and this loss indicates the presence of a tumour suppressor gene at this chromosomal location. This suppressor has turned out to be RB1.[15] About 50–70% of osteosarcomas have a hemizygous deletion affecting the RB1 gene,[16,17]

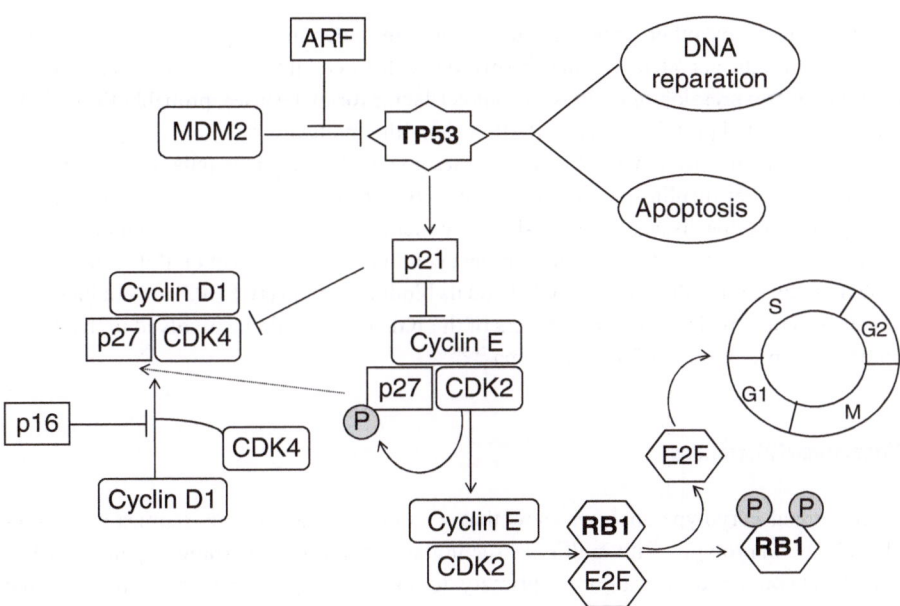

Fig. 2.1 Schematic representation of the cell cycle control mediated by TP53 and RB1

structural rearrangements (30%)[18] or point mutations of the gene (10%).[19] The presence of alterations at the RB1 locus can be considered an early marker of malignancy and of unfavourable prognosis and, in addition, RB1 alterations are more frequently encountered in high-grade than in low-grade osteosarcomas.[20,21] However, as with many of the molecular markers of this specific tumour, this prognostic association is not always found.[22]

Growth Factors

1. *Members of the WNT Family (Wingless-Type).* The WNT signalling pathway controls the normal bone formation during embryogenesis and bone homeostasis in the adult. The pathway has been investigated in the context of the osteosarcoma model in different publications. Recent data suggest that the WNT pathway may have a paracrine and autocrine effect involved in the metastatic potential of osteosarcoma,[23,24] although these data remain to be reproduced.
2. *Her-2/neu (Epidermal Growth Factor Receptor).* The overexpression of this tyrosine kinase is considered a poor prognostic factor in various types of carcinoma, since it is related with the tumour growth and the metastatic process. Even though the involvement of Her-2 in osteosarcoma has not been unequivocally established, and different reports show controversial results,[25,26] it is an attractive therapeutic target since an antagonist, Trastuzumab/Herceptin, is already available in the clinical setting.

There are many other genes of interest and are under investigation. One of these is *ezrin*, because the encoded protein is involved in cell-to-cell interaction and in signal transduction. Overexpression of ezrin is a promoter factor for metastases, probably through the mitogen-activated protein kinases (MAPK) signalling pathway.[27,28]

The fact that the peak incidence of osteosarcoma ovelaps with the pubertal growth spurt may indicate that insulin-like growth factor-I (*IGF-I*) and its receptor play a role in the pathogenesis of this disease. The IGF-I growth factor acts as a mitogen on both murine and human osteosarcoma cells, and osteosarcoma cell lines are dependent on IGF-I for in vitro growth. Even though the levels of IGF-I and its binding protein (IGFBP3) are not increased in osteosarcoma patients, other members of the IGF-I axis could be involved in the development and progression of osteosarcoma.[29,30]

Chromosomal Alterations

Conventional karyotype analyses show that, as a general rule, osteosarcomas have complex altered karyotypes with multiple structural and numerical aberrations. The most frequently encountered alterations in primary tumours (as opposed to cell lines) are the duplication of chromosome 1, loss of chromosomes 9, 10, 13 (RB1 locus) and 17 (TP53 locus), and either partial or complete loss of chromosome 6. The common findings of most cytogenetic studies indicate the presence of frequent breaks and aberrations at the following locations: 1p11-13, 1q11-12, 1q21-22, 11p15, 12p13, 17p11-13, 19q13 and 22q11-13.[31] Studies based on metaphase comparative genomic hybridization (CGH) have been a useful tool to unveil and characterise such complex karyotypes with high resolution and have identified high copy number regions or amplifications at 8q12-q21.3, 8q22-q23 (MYC gene) and at 17p11.2-17p12.[32] The chromosomal regions that are more frequently gained or lost have been carefully identified and reviewed.[33–35] Work by Ozaki and colleagues establishes that the gain or loss of some of these regions, either as isolated aberrations or as specific combinations, might have prognostic value.[36]

Ewing's Sarcoma Tumours

Introduction

Tumours within the Ewing's sarcoma family (EFTs) constitute the second most frequent type of bone-/soft-tissue sarcoma in children and adolescents.[37,38] The family comprises classical Ewing's sarcoma, peripheral primitive neuroectodermal tumours, and Askin's tumour, all of which are highly aggressive and frequently metastatic.[39] Tumours often appear in tubular bones of the appendicular skeleton (58%), although they also arise in the axial skeleton (33%) and at extraosseous sites.[40] Histologically, Ewing's tumours are characterised by the presence of small round cells with prominent and regular nuclei containing inconspicuous nucleoli, indistinct cytoplasm[38] and various degrees of neural and endothelial differentiation.[41]

Until the advent of differential molecular techniques, an unambiguous diagnosis required experienced pathological assessment. None of the markers used in conventional immunohistochemistry showed complete specificity. The transmembrane glycoprotein MIC2/CD99, the most specific marker so far, is expressed in more than 98% of EFTs.[42] Other tumours, including rabdomyosarcoma and lymphoblastic lymphoma, also present positive immunostaining. Depending on the degree of neuroectodermal differentiation, EFTs may also express neural markers, including S-100 synaptophysin, neural-specific enolase, CD57 and various neurofilaments.[43] The best tools for an unambiguous diagnosis are fluorescence in situ hybridisation and RT-PCR using a combination of primers targeting the underlying chromosomal translocations.[44]

Most of the progress over the last few decades has improved pathological definition and staging.[45] Despite a parallel improvement in treatment by multi-modal combination of surgery with chemo- and radio-therapy, the 5-year survival rate remains close to 50% for patients with primary tumours,[46] only 25% for patients with lung metastasis, and the prognosis for patients with bone or bone marrow metastasis is even worse.[47] The tumour also exhibits a strong tendency to metastasise through hematogenous spread to the lungs and frequently to the skeleton. Thus, in addition to the stage, location and size of the tumour, metastasis is a reliable prognosis factor indicative of poor prognosis.

Molecular Biology

The demonstration that fusion proteins are the "culprits" of the transforming events giving rise to hematological malignancies provided a strong rationale for investigation of fusion proteins in other tumours.

EFTs belong to a growing family of sarcomas characterised by specific reciprocal chromosomal translocations, which generate fusion genes: the neoplasm has a relatively simple cytogenetic background.[48]

At present, more than 15 different fusion proteins have been identified in EFTs. Chromosomal translocation t(11;22) q(24;q12) produces gene fusions between the amino terminus domain of EWS and the C-terminal region of a member belonging to the ETS family of transcription factors. Fusions resulting from the translocation give rise to functionally aberrant transcription factors potentially able to drive transformation in a permissive cellular context.

In 85% of Ewing's tumours, Friend Leukemia Integration 1 transcription factor (FLI-1) is the EWS partner which accounts for the different fusion subtypes observed.[49] Depending on the juxtaposed exons assembled by EWS and FLI-1 breakpoints, several subtypes have been described. Most tumours contain EWS/FLI-1 fusion types 1 (60%) and 2 (25%) which have been associated with different clinical features and prognosis.[50,51]

The FLI-1 gene displays a restricted pattern of expression, mainly in hematopoietic cells, and at lower levels in heart lung and ovaries.[52] During development FLI-1 is also expressed in neural crest-derived mesenchymal lineage and endothelial cells, which is consistent with its role in vasculogenesis and hematopoiesis.[53]

In contrast to FLI-1, the EWS gene encodes a ubiquitously expressed protein which belongs to the TET family of RNA binding proteins.[49,54] The TET family also includes TAFII68 (or TAF15)[55,56] and FUS (or TLS),[57] both of which share similar structural domains with EWS and have been found to form gene fusions with non-ETS transcription factors, giving rise to non-Ewing sarcomas such as myxoid liposarcomas,[58] myxoid chondrosarcomas[59] and desmoplastic small round-cell tumours,[60] with different histopathological features.

EWS contains three arginine–glycine–glycine (RGG) rich motifs that participate in RNA biogenesis and processing through interaction with proteins of the basal transcription machinery, including TFIID, RNA polymerase II[61,62] and coactivators such as CBP/p300.[55,54] In addition, TET proteins interact with splicing proteins. Indeed, EWS/FLI-1 has been shown to bind the splicing factor U1C and to modulate splicing activity.[62–64] Interaction with other proteins has also been described, for example, EWS interacts with BARD1, although the relevance of this to tumourogenesis has not been elucidated.[65]

Most studies have focused on the function of EWS as a transcription factor. The amino terminal domain of EWS contains a glutamine-rich N-terminal region containing a potent transcriptional activation domain[66,67] that, when fused to the DNA-binding domain of FLI-1, generates an aberrantly active transcription factor capable of specifically binding DNA.[68] Since the majority of fusion subtypes do not encompass the RGG domain, most studies have not assessed the effects of EWS–ETS fusions in RNA biogenesis.

All members of the ETS family of transcription factors are characterised by a common DNA-binding domain. Fusions of EWS with other ETS members have been described,[69] including ERG (in 10% of Ewing's tumours)[70] and with other fairly rare partners such as ETV1,[71] ETV4[72] and FEV.[73] The fact that different combinations of EWS/ETS give rise to Ewing's tumours of similar histopathology suggests that the potent transactivation domain of EWS, through interaction with other unknown proteins, is critical for transformation. Complementary to this view, the DNA binding domains of ETS proteins are highly homologous and all recognise targets containing a similar core sequence, and therefore, despite their differences, all EWS–ETS fusion proteins can be expected to act in a similar manner, disturbing a closely regulated pattern of gene transcription, with the consequent formation of Ewing's tumours.

The Oncoprotein EWS/FLI-1 as a Paradigm

The discovery of EWS/FLI-1 underscores the attractiveness of an approach to research looking to reveal common mechanisms in many tumours arising from specific translocations. Depending on the cellular background, EWS/FLI-1 induces a variety of responses that include transformation, senescence, differentiation, and cell lineage commitment.

The presence of neural markers and the diverse sites of origin have frequently led to the assumption or hypothesis that EFTs evolve from a cell type with multilineage differentiation potential.

In vitro experiments revealed that the chimeric EWS/FLI-1 acts as a potent repressor of normal cell fate. In murine primary marrow-derived stromal cells, EWS/FLI-1 represses osteogenic and adipogenic programs.[74,75] Similarly, myogenic differentiation was suppressed by the chimeric protein in a murine multipotent mesenchymal cell line.[74] In contrast, in other cellular backgrounds, EWS/FLI-1 dictates cell lineage commitment by redirecting cell lineage towards a neural-like phenotype.[76] Differentiation towards the neuroectodermal phenotype typical of Ewing's tumours, with the acquisition of a small round cell morphology, has been obtained in a fibroblastic cell line.[77] Similarly, in neuroblastoma, Hela, and rhabdomyosarcoma cell lines, the forced expression of EWS-FLI1 resulted in the acquisition of neural phenotypic traits.[78] Consistent with the role of FLI-1, in a separate rhabdomyosarcoma cell line, the expression of neural crest phenotypic markers was induced by EWS/FLI-1.[79]

In addition to repression of normal cell fate, EWS/FLI-1 is thought to induce cell-specific oncogenesis in a transformation-permissive cellular background. However, many cell lines, including Rat-1 fibroblasts, Ncm1, CTR, and the NIH 3T3-derived cell line YAL-7, have been found to be refractory to transformation.[80] Single-step oncogenesis has been reported in murine primary cells.[66,77,81,82] This finding can be attributed to a better transformation potential of rodent cells compared to human cells.[83,84] In the study by Castillero-Trejo et al, tumourogenicity increased with cell passage in culture and other secondary events, including p53 deletion.[81] These murine bone-derived cells expressing EWS/FLI-1 showed formation of sarcomatous tumours in syngeneic mice. Riggi et al reported that a single event of transduction with EWS/FLI-1 was sufficient to reconstitute the hallmarks of Ewing sarcomagenesis in a murine model.[82] In contrast, Riggi et al were unable to reproduce the same findings in primary human cells.[85] Studies of a human model have recently provided strong experimental evidence suggestive that the originating cell type is of mesenchymal lineage.[86]

In the mouse, background tumour suppressor pathways, including p16/p19 and p53, may be overcome by unknown factors. In human cells, however, additional mutations may be required to circumvent the strong tumour suppressor program. Indeed, other cytogenetic events[87] and additional mutations have been found in 20–30%[88–90] of human Ewing's tumours. An alternative suggestion recently put forward is that deregulated progenitor cells present in adult tissues are the cancer-initiating cells that are able to sustain tumour growth in vivo.[91,92] It is possible that the target for the transformation event driven by EWS/FLI-1 is an unidentified progenitor cell yet to be determined.

Target Genes

One of the main goals in the study of Ewing sarcomagenesis has been to identify downstream target genes regulated by EWS/FLI-1. Global transcriptomic analysis in combination with other techniques has elucidated several potential target genes involved in the genetic program driven by the fusion protein. The genes found are involved in neural differentiation, cell proliferation and anti-apoptotic functions. However, because the studies differ significantly depending on the chosen cellular model, it has been difficult to discern which EWS/FLI-1-responsive genes are associated with the initiation and maintenance of tumours.

The most compelling identification of a critical target of EWS/FLI-1 is that of the homeodomain protein NKX2.2.[93] NKX2.2 is transcriptional repressor involved in neural-cell differentiation. Induction of NKX2.2 is necessary for oncogenic transformation and represents a potential Ewing diagnostic marker. The protein's strong repressive function is mediated by a HDAC-dependent mechanism.[93,94]

Id2, a helix–loop–helix transcription factor without the DNA-binding domain, has been found to be upregulated by EWS/FLI-1 in Ewing's tumours. Through interaction with a variety of cell cycle proteins including p21 and Rb tumour suppressors,[95,96] Id2 is able to promote cell proliferation.

Other potential target genes transcriptionally upregulated by EWS/FLI-1 include PDGF-C,[97] which is expressed in more than 60% of tumours, CCND1[98,99] and c-Myc.[100,101]

hTERT, the catalytic subunit of telomerase and one of the hallmarks of many tumours, has also been found to be upregulated in approximately 80% of Ewing's samples. The upregulation is an indirect effect of EWS/FLI-1[102] through the recruitment of an unknown ancillary protein. Similarly, key tumour suppressors such as p57,[100] p21[103] and TGFBRII[104,105] were found to be downregulated in Ewing's tumours.

Interestingly, IGFBP-3 is a direct target of the fusion protein: EWS/FLI-1 binds to the IGFBP-3 promoter both in vitro and in vivo,[106] and the consequent repression leads to increased Akt activity and decreased apoptotic activity. Similarly, the IGF-1/IGF-1R axis, which is frequently required for Ewing's tumour cell growth, promotes cell survival through the Akt pathway.[107,108] Different pharmacological strategies targeting IGF1R are currently being explored for the treatment of Ewing's tumours.[109,110]

Recently, the combination of the techniques of transcriptomic analysis with high throughput chromatin immunoprecipitation analysis has validated previous research on EWS/FLI-1 by identifying previously reported genes (NKX2.2, ID2 and CCND1) and identifiying additional biologically relevant targets, including NROB1[111–113] and GAS1. The role of these targets in Ewing sarcomagenesis is yet to be determined.

Future Directions

The biology of EFTs remains an attractive experimental platform to understand critical questions regarding the development of both EFTs and a variety of other sarcomas. Despite the remarkable progress over the last two decades, there are still several questions that have not been rigorously addressed. Amongst these are the clear definition of the permissive cell and the specific time and microenvironment required for transformation. Similarly, the critical molecular events driven by the chimeric EWS/FLI-1 protein to initiate and maintain Ewing's tumours remain to be systematically dissected in an appropriate model. To this end, an animal model faithfully reproducing the spatio-temporal development of Ewing's sarcomas would be an invaluable tool. Only with precise knowledge at the cellular and molecular levels can we expect to elucidate critical target genes, and thereby facilitate the development of more focused and efficient therapies.

Referenes

1. Clark JC, Dass CR, Choong PF. A review of clinical and molecular prognostic factors in osteosarcoma. *J Cancer Res Clin Oncol*. 2008;134:281–297.
2. Ek ET, Ojaimi J, Kitagawa Y, Choong PF. Does the degree of intratumoral microvessel density and VEGF expression have prognostic significance in osteosarcoma. *Oncol Rep*. 2006;16:17–23.
3. Kreuter M, Bieker R, Bielack SS, et al. Prognostic relevance of increased angiogenesis in osteosarcoma. *Clin Cancer Res*. 2004;10:8531–8537.
4. Stempak D, Gammon J, Halton J, Moghrabi A, Koren G, Baruchel S. A pilot pharmacokinetic and antiangiogenic biomarker study of celecoxib and low-dose metronomic vinblastine or cyclophosphamide in pediatric recurrent solid tumors. *J Pediatr Hematol Oncol*. 2006;28:720–728.
5. Foukas AF, Deshmukh NS, Grimer RJ, Mangham DC, Mangos EG, Taylor S. Stage-IIB osteosarcomas around the knee A study of MMP-9 in surviving tumor cells. *J Bone Joint Surg Br*. 2002;84:706–711.
6. Kido A, Tsutsumi M, Iki K, et al. Overexpression of matrix metalloproteinase (MMP)-9 correlates with metastatic potency of spontaneous and 4-hydroxyaminoquinoline 1-oxide (4-HAQO)-induced transplantable osteosarcomas in rats. *Cancer Lett*. 1999;137:209–216.
7. Pakos EE, Ioannidis JP. The association of P-glycoprotein with response to chemotherapy and clinical outcome in patients with osteosarcoma A meta-analysis. *Cancer*. 2003 August 1;98(3): 581–589.
8. Baldini N, Scotlandi K, Serra M, et al. P-glycoprotein expression in osteosarcoma: a basis for risk-adapted adjuvant chemotherapy. *J Orthop Res*. 1999;17:629–632.
9. Park YB, Kim HS, Oh JH, Lee SH. The co-expression of p53 protein and P-glycoprotein is correlated to a poor prognosis in osteosarcoma. *Int Orthop*. 2001;24:307–310.
10. Kansara M, Thomas DM. Molecular pathogenesis of osteosarcoma. *DNA Cell Biol*. 2007;26:1–18.

11. Soussi T, Leblanc T, Baruchel A, Schaison G. Germline mutations of the p53 tumor-suppressor gene in cancer-prone families: a review. *Nouv Rev Fr Hematol*. 1993;35:33–36.

12. Kaseta MK, Khaldi L, Gomatos IP, et al. Prognostic value of bax, bcl-2, and p53 staining in primary osteosarcoma. *J Surg Oncol*. 2008;97:259–266.

13. Wunder JS, Gokgoz N, Parkes R, et al. TP53 mutations and outcome in osteosarcoma: a prospective, multicenter study. *J Clin Oncol*. 2005;23:1483–1490.

14. Belchis DA, Gocke CD, Geradts J. Alterations in the rb, p16, and cyclin d1 cell cycle control pathway in osteosarcomas. *Pediat Pathol Mol Med*. 2000;19:377–389.

15. Yamaguchi T, Toguchida J, Yamamuro T, et al. Allelotype analysis in osteosarcomas: frequent allele loss on 3q, 13q, 17p, and 18q. *Cancer Res*. 1992;52:2419–2423.

16. Wadayama B, Feugeas O, Guriec N, et al. Loss of heterozygosity of the RB gene is a poor prognostic factor in patients with osteosarcoma. *J Clin Oncol*. 1996;14:467–472.

17. Benassi MS, Molendini L, Gamberi G, et al. Alteration of pRb/p16/cdk4 regulation in human osteosarcoma. *Int J Cancer*. 1999;84:489–493.

18. Miller CW, Aslo A, Won A, Tan M, Lampkin B, Koeffler HP. Alterations of the p53, Rb and MDM2 genes in osteosarcoma. *J Cancer Res Clin Oncol*. 1996;122:559–565.

19. Wadayama B, Toguchida J, Shimizu T, et al. Mutation spectrum of the retinoblastoma gene in osteosarcomas. *Cancer Res*. 1994;54:3042–3048.

20. Patiño-García A, Piñeiro ES, Díez MZ, Iturriagagoitia LG, Klüssmann FA, Ariznabarreta LS. Genetic and epigenetic alterations of the cell cycle regulators and tumor suppressor genes in pediatric osteosarcomas. *J Pediatr Hematol Oncol*. 2003;25:362–367.

21. Wunder JS, Czitrom AA, Kandel R, Andrulis IL. Analysis of alterations in the retinoblastoma gene and tumor grade in bone and soft-tissue sarcomas. *J Natl Cancer Inst*. 1991;83: 194–200.

22. Heinsohn S, Evermann U, Zur Stadt U, Bielack S, Kabisch H. Determination of the prognostic value of loss of heterozygosity at the retinoblastoma gene in osteosarcoma. *Int J Oncol*. 2007;30:1205–1214.

23. Chen K, Fallen S, Abaan HO, Hayran M, et al. WNT10b induces chemotaxis of osteosarcoma and correlates with reduced survival. *Pediatr Blood Cancer*. 2008;51:349–355.

24. Hoang BH, Kubo T, Healey JH, et al. Expression of LDL receptor-related protein 5 (LRP5) as a novel marker for disease progression in high-grade osteosarcoma. *Int J Cancer*. 2004; 109:106–111.

25. Rakesh Kumar V, Gupta N, Kakkar N, Sharma SC. Prognostic and predictive value of c-erbB2 overexpression in osteogenic sarcoma. *J Cancer Res Ther*. 2006;2:20–23.

26. Zhou H, Randall RL, Brothman AR, Maxwell T, Coffin CM, Goldsby RE. Her-2/neu expression in osteosarcoma increases risk of lung metastasis and can be associated with gene amplification. *J Pediatr Hematol Oncol*. 2003;25:27–32.

27. Ferrari S, Zanella L, Alberghini M, Palmerini E, Staals E, Bacchini P. Prognostic significance of immunohistochemical expression of ezrin in non-metastatic high-grade osteosarcoma. *Pediatr Blood Cancer*. 2008;50:752–756.

28. Park HR, Jung WW, Bacchini P, Bertoni F, Kim YW, Park YK. Ezrin in osteosarcoma: comparison between conventional high-grade and central low-grade osteosarcoma. *Pathol Res Pract*. 2006;202:509–515.

29. Chavez Kappel C, Velez-Yanguas C, Hirschfeld S, Helman LJ. Human osteosarcoma cell lines are dependent on insulin-like growth factor for in vitro growth. *Cancer Res*. 1994; 54:2803–2807.

30. Rodriguez-Galindo C, Poquette CA, Daw NC, Tan M, Meyer WH, and Cleveland JL. Circulating concentrations of IGF-I and IGFBP-3 are not predictive of incidence or clinical behavior of pediatric osteosarcoma. *Med Pediatr Oncol*. 2001;36:605–611.

31. Sandberg AA, Bridge JA. Updates on the cytogenetics and molecular genetics of bone and soft tissue tumors: osteosarcoma and related tumors. *Cancer Genet Cytogenet*. 2003;145:1–30.

32. Squire JA, Pei J, Marrano P, et al. High-resolution mapping of amplifications and deletions in pediatric osteosarcoma by use of CGH analysis of cDNA microarrays. *Genes Chromosomes Cancer*. 2003;38:215–225.

33. Forus A, Weghuis DO, Smeets D, Fodstad O, Myklebost O, Geurts van Kessel A. Comparative genomic hybridization analysis of human sarcomas: II. Identification of novel amplicons at 6p and 17p in osteosarcomas. *Genes Chromosomes Cancer*. 1995;14:15–21.

34. Tarkkanen M, Karhu R, Kallioniemi A, et al. Gains and losses of DNA sequences in osteosarcomas by comparative genomic hybridization. *Cancer Res*. 1995;55:1334–1338.

35. Zielenska M, Marrano P, Thorner P, et al. High-resolution cDNA microarray CGH mapping of genomic imbalances in osteosarcoma using formalin-fixed paraffin-embedded tissue. *Cytogenet Genome Res*. 2004;107:77–82.

36. Ozaki T, Schaefer KL, Wai D, et al. Genetic imbalances revealed by comparative genomic hybridization in osteosarcomas. *Int J Cancer*. 2002;102:355–365.

37. Gurney JG, Davis S, Severson RK, Fang JY, Ross JA, Robison LL. Trends in cancer incidence among children in the U.S. *Cancer*. 1996;78:532–541.

38. Arndt CA, Crist WM. Common musculoskeletal tumors of childhood and adolescence. *N Engl J Med*. 1999;341:342–352.

39. de Alava E, Gerald WL. Molecular biology of the Ewing's sarcoma/primitive neuroectodermal tumor family. *J Clin Oncol*. 2000;18:204–213.

40. Grier HE. The Ewing family of tumors Ewing's sarcoma and primitive neuroectodermal tumors. *Pediatr Clin North Am*. 1997;44:991–1004.

41. Franchi A, Pasquinelli G, Cenacchi G, et al. Immunohistochemical and ultrastructural investigation of neural differentiation in Ewing sarcoma/PNET of bone and soft tissues. *Ultrastruct Pathol*. 2001;25:219–225.

42. Kovar H, Dworzak M, Strehl S, et al. Overexpression of the pseudoautosomal gene MIC2 in Ewing's sarcoma and peripheral primitive neuroectodermal tumor. *Oncogene*. 1990;5:1067–1070.

43. Ushigome SMR, Sorensen PH. Ewing sarcoma/Primitive neuroectodermal tumor (PNET). In: Christopher DM, Fletcher KKU, Fredrik M, eds. *Pathology and Genetics of Tumors of Soft Tissue and Bone World Health Organization Classification of Tumors*. Lyon: Pathology and Genetics of Tumors of Soft Tissue and Bone International Agency for Research on Cancer; 2002.

44. Peter M, Gilbert E, Delattre O. A multiplex real-time PCR assay for the detection of gene fusions observed in solid tumors. *Lab Invest*. 2001;81:905–912.

45. Burchill SA. Ewing's sarcoma: diagnostic, prognostic, and therapeutic implications of molecular abnormalities. *J Clin Pathol*. 2003;56:96–102.

46. Paulussen M, Ahrens S, Craft AW, et al. Ewing's tumors with primary lung metastases: survival analysis of 114 (European Intergroup) Cooperative Ewing's Sarcoma Studies patients. *J Clin Oncol*. 1998;16:3044–3052.

47. Cotterill SJ, Ahrens S, Paulussen M, et al. Prognostic factors in Ewing's tumor of bone: analysis of 975 patients from the European Intergroup Cooperative Ewing's Sarcoma Study Group. *J Clin Oncol*. 2000;18:3108–114.

48. Mackall CL, Meltzer PS, Helman LJ. Focus on sarcomas. *Cancer Cell*. 2002;2:175–178.

49. Delattre O, Zucman J, Plougastel B, et al. Gene fusion with an ETS DNA-binding domain caused by chromosome translocation in human tumors. *Nature*. 1992;359:162–165.

50. de Alava E, Kawai A, Healey JH, et al. EWS-FLI1 fusion transcript structure is an independent determinant of prognosis in Ewing's sarcoma. *J Clin Oncol*. 1998;16:1248–1255.

51. Zoubek A, Dockhorn-Dworniczak B, Delattre O, et al. Does expression of different EWS chimeric transcripts define clinically distinct risk groups of Ewing tumor patients. *J. Clin Oncol*. 1996;14:1245–1251.

52. Ben-David Y, Giddens EB, Letwin K, Bernstein A. Erythroleukemia induction by Friend murine leukemia virus: insertional activation of a new member of the ets gene family, Fli-1, closely linked to c-ets-1. *Genes Dev*. 1991;5:908–918.

53. Melet F, Motro B, Rossi DJ, Zhang L, Bernstein A. Generation of a novel Fli-1 protein by gene targeting leads to a defect in thymus development and a delay in Friend virus-induced erythroleukemia. *Mol Cell Biol.* 1996;16:2708–2718.

54. Ohno T, Ouchida M, Lee L, Gatalica Z, Rao VN, Reddy ES. The EWS gene, involved in Ewing family of tumors, malignant melanoma of soft parts and desmoplastic small round cell tumors, codes for an RNA binding protein with novel regulatory domains. *Oncogene.* 1994;9: 3087–3097.

55. Bertolotti A, Lutz Y, Heard DJ, Chambon P, Tora L. hTAF(II)68, a novel RNA/ssDNA-binding protein with homology to the pro-oncoproteins TLS/FUS and EWS is associated with both TFIID and RNA polymerase II. *EMBO J.* 1996;15:5022–5031.

56. Aman P, Panagopoulos I, Lassen C, et al. Expression patterns of the human sarcoma-associated genes FUS and EWS and the genomic structure of FUS. *Genomics.* 1996;37:1–8.

57. Shing DC, McMullan DJ, Roberts P, et al. FUS/ERG gene fusions in Ewing's tumors. *Cancer Res.* 2003;63:4568–4576.

58. Crozat A, Aman P, Mandahl N, Ron D. Fusion of CHOP to a novel RNA-binding protein in human myxoid liposarcoma. *Nature.* 1993;363:640–644.

59. Labelle Y, Zucman J, Stenman G, et al. Oncogenic conversion of a novel orphan nuclear receptor by chromosome translocation. *Hum Mol Genet.* 1995;4:2219–2226.

60. Ladanyi M, Gerald W. Fusion of the EWS and WT1 genes in the desmoplastic small round cell tumor. *Cancer Res.* 1994;54:2837–2840.

61. Petermann R, Mossier BM, Aryee DN, Khazak V, Golemis EA, Kovar H. Oncogenic EWS-Fli1 interacts with hsRPB7, a subunit of human RNA polymerase II. *Oncogene.* 1998;17:603–610.

62. Yang L, Chansky HA, Hickstein DD. EWS.Fli-1 fusion protein interacts with hyperphospho-rylated RNA polymerase II and interferes with serine-arginine protein-mediated RNA splicing. *J Biol Chem.* 2000;275:37612–37618.

63. Knoop LL, Baker SJ. The splicing factor U1C represses EWS/FLI-mediated transactivation. *J Biol Chem.* 2000;275:24865–24871.

64. Knoop LL, Baker SJ. EWS/FLI alters 5''-splice site selection. *J Biol Chem.* 2001; 276:22317–22322.

65. Spahn L, Petermann R, Siligan C, Schmid JA, Aryee DN, Kovar H. Interaction of the EWS NH2 terminus with BARD1 links the Ewing's sarcoma gene to a common tumor suppressor pathway. *Cancer Res.* 2002;62:4583–4587.

66. May WA, Gishizky ML, Lessnick SL, et al. Ewing sarcoma 11;22 translocation produces a chimeric transcription factor that requires the DNA-binding domain encoded by FLI1 for transformation. *Proc Natl Acad Sci U S A.* 1993;90:5752–5756.

67. Lessnick SL, Braun BS, Denny CT, May WA. Multiple domains mediate transformation by the Ewing's sarcoma EWS/FLI-1 fusion gene. *Oncogene.* 1995;10:423–431.

68. Janknecht R, Nordheim A. Gene regulation by Ets proteins. *Biochim Biophys Acta.* 1993; 1155:346–356.

69. Huang HY, Illei PB, Zhao Z, et al. Ewing sarcomas with p53 mutation or p16/p14ARF homozygous deletion: a highly lethal subset associated with poor chemoresponse. *J Clin Oncol.* 2005;23:548–558.

70. Zucman J, Melot T, Desmaze C, et al. Combinatorial generation of variable fusion proteins in the Ewing family of tumors. *EMBO J.* 1993;12:4481–4487.

71. Jeon IS, Davis JN, Braun BS, et al. A variant Ewing's sarcoma translocation (7;22) fuses the EWS gene to the ETS gene ETV1. *Oncogene.* 1995;10:1229–1234.

72. Kaneko Y, Yoshida K, Handa M, et al. Fusion of an ETS-family gene, EIAF, to EWS by t(17;22)(q12;q12) chromosome translocation in an undifferentiated sarcoma of infancy. *Genes Chromosomes Cancer.* 1996;15:115–121.

73. Peter M, Couturier J, Pacquement H, et al. A new member of the ETS family fused to EWS in Ewing tumors. *Oncogene.* 1997;14:1159–1164.

74. Torchia EC, Jaishankar S, Baker SJ. Ewing tumor fusion proteins block the differentiation of pluripotent marrow stromal cells. *Cancer Res.* 2003;63:3464–3468.

75. Gonzalez I, Vicent S, de Alava E, Lecanda F. EWS/FLI-1 oncoprotein subtypes impose different requirements for transformation and metastatic activity in a murine model. *J Mol Med.* 2007;85:1015–1029.

76. Gershon TR, Oppenheimer O, Chin SS, Gerald WL. Temporally regulated neural crest transcription factors distinguish neuroectodermal tumors of varying malignancy and differentiation. *Neoplasia.* 2005;7:575–584.

77. Teitell MA, Thompson AD, Sorensen PH, Shimada H, Triche TJ, Denny CT. EWS/ETS fusion genes induce epithelial and neuroectodermal differentiation in NIH 3T3 fibroblasts. *Lab Invest.* 1999;79:1535–1543.

78. Rorie CJ, Thomas VD, Chen P, Pierce HH, O'Bryan JP, Weissman BE. The Ews/Fli-1 fusion gene switches the differentiation program of neuroblastomas to Ewing sarcoma/peripheral primitive neuroectodermal tumors. *Cancer Res.* 2004;64:1266–1277.

79. Hu-Lieskovan S, Zhang J, Wu L, Shimada H, Schofield DE, Triche TJ. EWS-FLI1 fusion protein up-regulates critical genes in neural crest development and is responsible for the observed phenotype of Ewing's family of tumors. *Cancer Res.* 2005;65:4633–4644.

80. Deneen B, Denny CT. Loss of p16 pathways stabilizes EWS/FLI1 expression and complements EWS/FLI1 mediated transformation. *Oncogene.* 2001;20:6731–6741.

81. Castillero-Trejo Y, Eliazer S, Xiang L, Richardson JA, Ilaria RL, Jr. Expression of the EWS/FLI-1 oncogene in murine primary bone-derived cells results in EWS/FLI-1-dependent, Ewing sarcoma-like tumors. *Cancer Res.* 2005;65:8698–8705.

82. Riggi N, Cironi L, Provero P, et al. Development of Ewing's sarcoma from primary bone marrow-derived mesenchymal progenitor cells. *Cancer Res.* 2005;65:11459–11468.

83. Tolar J, Nauta AJ, Osborn MJ, et al. Sarcoma derived from cultured mesenchymal stem cells. *Stem Cells.* 2007;25:371–379.

84. Rangarajan A, Hong SJ, Gifford A, Weinberg RA. Species- and cell type-specific requirements for cellular transformation. *Cancer Cell.* 2004;6:171–183.

85. Riggi N, Suva ML, Suva D, et al. EWS-FLI-1 expression triggers a Ewing's sarcoma initiation program in primary human mesenchymal stem cells. *Cancer Res.* 2008;68:2176–2185.

86. Tirode F, Laud-Duval K, Prieur A, Delorme B, Charbord P, Delattre O. Mesenchymal stem cell features of Ewing tumors. *Cancer Cell.* 2007;11:421–429.

87. Szuhai K, Ijszenga M, Tanke HJ, Rosenberg C, Hogendoorn PC. Molecular cytogenetic characterization of four previously established and two newly established Ewing sarcoma cell lines. *Cancer Genet Cytogenet.* 2006;166:173–179.

88. Kovar H, Jug G, Aryee DN, et al. Among genes involved in the RB dependent cell cycle regulatory cascade, the p16 tumor suppressor gene is frequently lost in the Ewing family of tumors. Oncogene. 1997;15:2225–2232.

89. Tsuchiya T, Sekine K, Hinohara S, Namiki T, Nobori T, Kaneko Y. Analysis of the p16INK4, p14ARF, p15, TP53, and MDM2 genes and their prognostic implications in osteosarcoma and Ewing sarcoma. Cancer Genet Cytogenet. 2000;120:91–98.

90. Lopez-Guerrero JA, Pellin A, Noguera R, Carda C, Llombart-Bosch A. Molecular analysis of the 9p21 locus and p53 genes in Ewing family tumors. Lab Invest. 2001;81:803–814.

91. Bonnet D, Dick JE. Human acute myeloid leukemia is organized as a hierarchy that originates from a primitive hematopoietic cell. Nat Med. 1997;3:730–737.

92. Jamieson CH, Weissman IL, Passegue E. Chronic versus acute myelogenous leukemia: a question of self-renewal. Cancer Cell. 2004;6:531–533.

93. Smith R, Owen LA, Trem DJ, et al. Expression profiling of EWS/FLI identifies NKX2.2 as a critical target gene in Ewing's sarcoma. Cancer Cell. 2006;9:405–416.

94. Owen LA, Kowalewski AA, Lessnick SL. EWS/FLI mediates transcriptional repression via NKX2.2 during oncogenic transformation in Ewing's sarcoma. PLoS ONE. 2008;3:e1965.

95. Fukuma M, Okita H, Hata J, Umezawa A. Upregulation of Id2, an oncogenic helix-loop-helix protein, is mediated by the chimeric EWS/ets protein in Ewing sarcoma. *Oncogene.* 2003;22:1–9.

96. Nishimori H, Sasaki Y, Yoshida K, et al. The Id2 gene is a novel target of transcriptional activation by EWS-ETS fusion proteins in Ewing family tumors. *Oncogene.* 2002;21:8302–8309.

97. Zwerner JP, May WA. PDGF-C is an EWS/FLI induced transforming growth factor in Ewing family tumors. *Oncogene.* 2001;20:626–633.

98. Matsumoto Y, Tanaka K, Nakatani F, Matsunobu T, Matsuda S, Iwamoto Y. Downregulation and forced expression of EWS-Fli1 fusion gene results in changes in the expression of G(1) regulatory genes. *Br J Cancer.* 2001;84:768–775.

99. Wai DH, Schaefer KL, Schramm A, et al. Expression analysis of pediatric solid tumor cell lines using oligonucleotide microarrays. *Int J Oncol.* 2002;20:441–451.

100. Dauphinot L, De Oliveira C, Melot T, et al. Analysis of the expression of cell cycle regulators in Ewing cell lines: EWS-FLI-1 modulates p57KIP2and c-Myc expression. *Oncogene.* 2001;20:3258–3265.

101. Bailly RA, Bosselut R, Zucman J, et al. DNA-binding and transcriptional activation properties of the EWS-FLI-1 fusion protein resulting from the t(11;22) translocation in Ewing sarcoma. *Mol Cell Biol.* 1994;14:3230–3241.

102. Takahashi A, Higashino F, Aoyagi M, et al. EWS/ETS fusions activate telomerase in Ewing's tumors. *Cancer Res.* 2003;63:8338–8344.

103. Nakatani F, Tanaka K, Sakimura R, et al. Identification of p21WAF1/CIP1 as a direct target of EWS-Fli1 oncogenic fusion protein. *J Biol Chem.* 2003;278:15105–15115.

104. Hahm KB. Repression of the gene encoding the TGF-beta type II receptor is a major target of the EWS-FLI1 oncoprotein. *Nat Genet.* 1999;23:481.

105. Im YH, Kim HT, Lee C, et al. EWS-FLI1, EWS-ERG, and EWS-ETV1 oncoproteins of Ewing tumor family all suppress transcription of transforming growth factor beta type II receptor gene. *Cancer Res.* 2000;60:1536–1540.

106. Prieur A, Tirode F, Cohen P, Delattre O. EWS/FLI-1 silencing and gene profiling of Ewing cells reveal downstream oncogenic pathways and a crucial role for repression of insulin-like growth factor binding protein 3. *Mol Cell Biol.* 2004;24:7275–7283.

107. Scotlandi K, Benini S, Nanni P, et al. Blockage of insulin-like growth factor-I receptor inhibits the growth of Ewing's sarcoma in athymic mice. *Cancer Res.* 1998;58:4127–4131.

108. Scotlandi K, Avnet S, Benini S, et al. Expression of an IGF-I receptor dominant negative mutant induces apoptosis, inhibits tumorigenesis and enhances chemosensitivity in Ewing's sarcoma cells. *Int J Cancer.* 2002;101:11–16.

109. Scotlandi K, Maini C, Manara MC, et al. Effectiveness of insulin-like growth factor I receptor antisense strategy against Ewing's sarcoma cells. *Cancer Gene Ther.* 2002;9:296–307.

110. Manara MC, Landuzzi L, Nanni P, et al. Preclinical in vivo study of new insulin-like growth factor-I receptor-specific inhibitor in Ewing's sarcoma. *Clin Cancer Res.* 2007;13:1322–1330.

111. Kinsey M, Smith R, Lessnick SL. NR0B1 is required for the oncogenic phenotype mediated by EWS/FLI in Ewing's sarcoma. *Mol Cancer Res.* 2006;4:851–859.

112. Garcia-Aragoncillo E, Carrillo J, Lalli E, et al. DAX1, a direct target of EWS/FLI1 oncoprotein, is a principal regulator of cell-cycle progression in Ewing's tumor cells. *Oncogene.* 2008.

113. Mendiola M, Carrillo J, Garcia E, et al. The orphan nuclear receptor DAX1 is up-regulated by the EWS/FLI1 oncoprotein and is highly expressed in Ewing tumors. *Int J Cancer.* 2006;118:1381–1389.

Surgical Options for Limb Salvage in Immature Patients with Extremity Sarcoma

3

Mathew J. Most and Franklin H. Sim

Abstract The different types of limb salvage procedures can be classified as biologic (i.e. autograft, allograft), non-biologic (i.e. megaprosthesis, expandable prosthesis), or combination (i.e. allograft-prosthetic composite). Each of these types has its own indications, as well as advantages and disadvantages.

Introduction

Primary bone and soft tissue sarcomas are rare in children. In the USA, the average annual incidence of cancer of the bone in children under the age of 20 is 8.7 per million. This amounts to approximately 650–700 new malignant bone tumours per year in children and adolescents. Almost two-thirds of these cases are of osteogenic sarcoma, and most of the remaining one-third are cases of Ewing's sarcoma.[20] Overall, these cases account for 6% of all paediatric malignancies.[24]

Over the last 30–40 years, great advances have been made in the diagnosis and treatment of these conditions. Improvements in imaging, chemotherapy, and surgical technique have increased 5-year survival from historical rates of 10–20% to current rates of 60–70%.[3,43] This, in turn, has led to increasing interest in preserving a functional limb for the patient.[30,43] Thirty years ago, approximately 80% of paediatric patients with an extremity sarcoma would have been treated with an amputation. Now, 80–90% of patients can undergo a limb-sparing procedure.[24,28]

General Considerations

Limb salvage surgery in the paediatric population presents unique challenges. These include the smaller size of a young patient's skeleton, the growth potential of the unaffected leg and eventual limb-length discrepancy, and the need for a durable reconstruction that can withstand the high activity levels and long-life expectancies in these younger patients.[29]

Mathew J. Most (✉)
Department of Orthopedic Surgery, Mayo Clinic, 200 First Street SW, Rochester, MN, USA
e-mail: mathewjmost@hotmail.com

J. Cañadell and M. San-Julian (eds.), *Pediatric Bone Sarcomas: Epiphysiolysis Before Excision*,
DOI: 10.1007/978-1-84882-130-9_3, © Springer-Verlag London Limited 2011

The most common locations for these malignant bone lesions include the distal femur, proximal tibia, and proximal humerus; approximately 75% of these tumours occur near a physis.[10] Resection of these tumours therefore often entails excision of the physis (or multiple physes) as well, which can have a significant effect on the remaining growth of the salvaged extremity. In the lower extremity, 60–70% of limb growth occurs around the knee (distal femoral and proximal tibial physes), and 80% of the growth of the humerus occurs at the proximal physis.[1,4] As such, after treatment of these tumours, a significant limb-length discrepancy can develop.

Leg-length discrepancies of less than 2 cm in the lower extremities are well-tolerated, with little to no functional or clinical significance. These can often be treated with shoe modifications (i.e. shoe lifts) alone. If a predicted limb-length discrepancy will be less than 2 cm, the affected leg can be slightly over-lengthened by a centimetre or so at resection and reconstruction to compensate as well. In the still-growing child, predicted discrepancies of 2–4 cm can usually be treated with epiphysiodesis of the contralateral extremity or lengthening procedures on the involved side. However, predicted leg-length differences of greater than 4 cm generally require other types of procedures, and often multiple interventions, to achieve similar ultimate limb lengths.[16,29]

Therefore, a relative contraindication to limb-sparing surgery is very immature skeletal age (<8 years old). A patient this young would have a very large anticipated limb-length discrepancy, likely requiring multiple operations over many years to minimize the length difference, with each procedure entailing the inherent risks of surgery.[43] However, San-Julian and colleagues reported on a series of 40 patients under the age of 10 treated with physeal-sparing limb salvage for extremity sarcoma. Their overall survival rate was 75% at final follow-up, with 90% of the patients retaining their extremity.[40] Moreover, newer expandable prostheses, which do not require surgery or anaesthesia to lengthen, may facilitate limb salvage in this age group.

Types of Limb Salvage Procedures

The types of limb salvage procedures can be classified as biologic (i.e. autograft, allograft), non-biologic (i.e. megaprosthesis, expandable prosthesis), or combination (i.e. allograft-prosthetic composite).[1] Each of these types has its own indications, as well as advantages and disadvantages.

Biological Reconstruction

Biological reconstructions utilize autograft and/or allograft bone to fill in defects subsequent to tumour resection, and rely on bone to bone healing for ultimate stability. For metadiaphyseal tumours, often an intercalary resection and reconstruction can be performed (allograft, autograft, or combination), salvaging the joints above and below the tumour. If the tumour encroaches upon or involves the joint, then osteoarticular allograft remains an option for biological reconstruction.

Another important consideration is the location of the tumour relative to the physes of the involved bone. If the tumour resection involves removal of one or more physes, then limb-length discrepancy can be problematic if significant skeletal growth potential remains. This may have to be addressed with lengthening procedures on the involved side and/or epiphysiodesis or shortening procedures on the contralateral extremity.

Intercalary Allografts

Massive allografts have a long history of use in reconstruction after tumour resection in adult patients, with generally good results. A long-term study of 104 intercalary allograft procedures performed at the Massachusetts General Hospital (adult and children) and published in 1997 reported an overall success rate of 84% at an average follow-up of 5.6 years[38] (Figs. 3.1 and 3.2).

In 1995, Alman and colleagues reported a review of 26 paediatric and adolescent patients who underwent tumour resection and massive allograft reconstruction. Eighteen of the 26 patients had an excellent or good result at final follow-up, and 88% of patients with a lower extremity reconstruction that survived their disease retained their allograft at

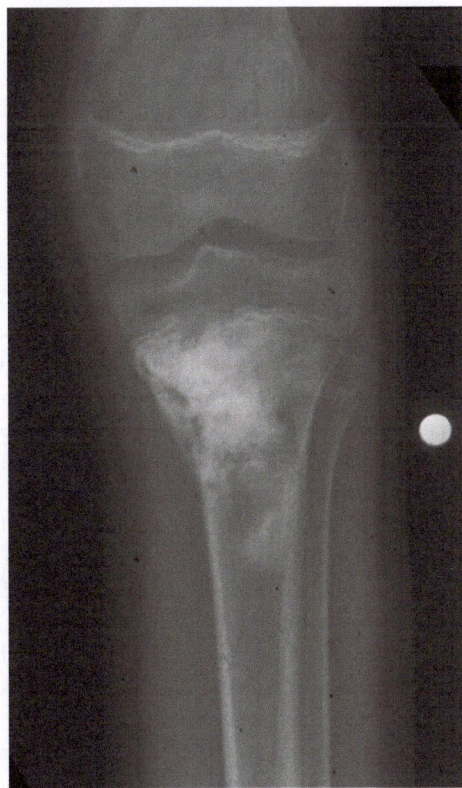

Fig. 3.1 Anteroposterior (*AP*) radiograph of the knee, demonstrating osteosarcoma of the proximal tibia in an 11-year-old

Fig. 3.2 The same patient, as in Fig. 3.1, following resection of the proximal tibial osteosarcoma and reconstruction with an osteoarticular allograft

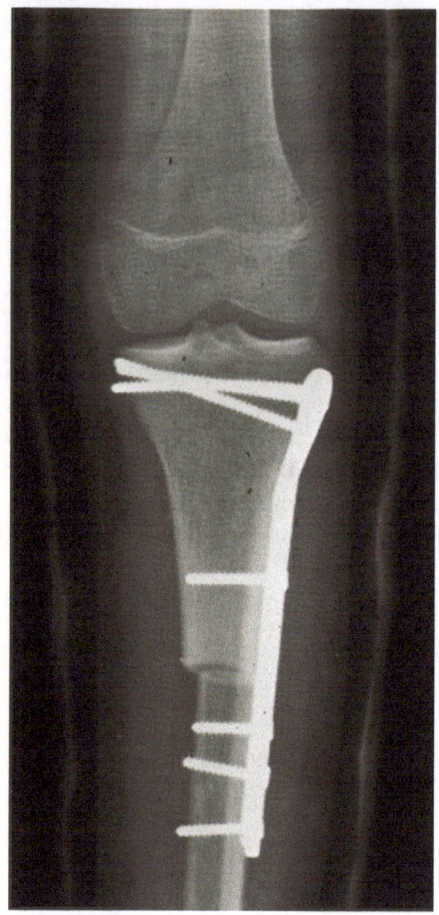

final follow-up. However, complication rates were high. At least one complication occurred in 77% of the patients (not including limb-length discrepancy). Allograft fractures occurred in 54%, and the infection rate was 12%. Two of the three patients who developed infection went on to amputation. Four patients (15%) developed a non-union; each was treated with an additional autologous bone grafting procedure, and each went on to heal within 12 months. A limb-length discrepancy over 2 cm occurred in 60% of patients with lower extremity reconstruction. The authors concluded that, although the complication rate was higher than in adults, allograft reconstruction was a useful option in younger patients in whom limb-length discrepancy would be predicted to be mild, or those discrepancies that could be easily treated.[2]

More recently, Musculo and colleagues published a series of 22 patients under the age of 10 who had massive allografts placed after sarcoma resection (13 intercalary and 9 osteoarticular). At latest follow-up, 3 patients died of their disease, 1 patient had a subsequent amputation, and 18 patients were alive and had retained their limb. Fifteen of those 18 retained their original allograft. Eight complications occurred which required repeat surgeries (three local recurrences, three fractures, one infection, and one non-union); four of the eight had their original allograft preserved. Mean Musculoskeletal Tumour Society (MSTS) functional scores and International Society of Limb Salvage radiographic scores were 27% and 94%, respectively. Four patients that had both physes preserved had no limb-length discrepancy at final follow-up. Fourteen patients that had resection of one physis with their tumour had a mean leg-length discrepancy of 2.1 cm at latest follow-up. The authors therefore concluded that allograft reconstruction was an acceptable technique in young children with extremity sarcoma.[34]

Osteoarticular Allografts

Osteoarticular allografts tend to do less well than intercalary allografts, and this is generally due to degeneration of the allograft articular surface secondary to chondrocyte cell death and subchondral bone resorption and collapse.[21,32] Musculo and colleagues reported on a series of 76 adult and paediatric patients with a tumour of the distal femur that underwent a resection and reconstruction with a distal femoral osteoarticular allograft. Overall allograft survival was 78% at both 5 and 10 years, and the rate of allograft survival without the need for joint resurfacing was 71% at both 5 and 10 years. However, 35% of patients did have radiographic evidence of joint degeneration.[35]

In another large series of osteoarticular allografts, Mnaymneh and co-authors reported on a series of 96 patients (adult and paediatric) who underwent distal femoral osteoarticular allograft reconstruction after resection of benign or malignant tumours. Overall complications included a fracture rate of 14%, non-union rate of 12%, and infection rate of 6%. Clinically significant arthritis developed in 10%, and instability in 7%. Significant differences were seen in the results based upon whether or not the patient had received chemotherapy. The overall complication rate in the chemotherapy group was 47%, compared to 30% in those patients who did not undergo chemotherapy. In patients who had received chemotherapy, the infection rate was 13% (vs 2% without chemotherapy), and the non-union rate was 23% (vs 6%). The modified Mankin classification system was utilized to grade the functional results. Of the patients who did not receive chemotherapy, 70% had good or excellent results, 26% had fair results, and 4% had poor results. In contrast, for those patients who underwent chemotherapy, only 53% had good or excellent results, 37% had fair results, and 10% had poor results. Although the complication rates were high, the authors felt that osteoarticular allograft reconstruction was a viable option, in which most of the complications could be treated adequately.[32]

Autografts

While the aforementioned studies, and others, show that massive allografts are useful in paediatric bone sarcoma reconstructions, these procedures are associated with relatively high complication rates. The three most common complications associated with massive allograft reconstruction include infection, non-union, and fracture. These complications are likely related to the avascular status of the allograft bone.[33] In an effort to reduce these

complication rates, free vascularized fibula autografts have been used to reconstruct segmental defects after sarcoma resection. The vascularized fibula graft brings well-perfused
bone to the site that is capable of osteogenesis. However, being of smaller diameter, it usually lacks the mechanical strength of large allografts. The fibular autograft will grow,
hypertrophy, and remodel over time, but this takes a considerable amount of time, and
repeated stress fractures may require repetitive prolonged immobilization.[33]

Chen and colleagues from the Memorial Sloan Kettering Cancer Centre reported on a
series of 25 consecutive patients (adult and paediatric) treated with a vascularized fibular
free flap after limb-sparing resection of extremity sarcomas. All flaps survived to final
follow-up. The infection rate was 12%. Uncomplicated bony union occurred in 78% within
6 months. After secondary bone grafting procedures, 93% ultimately went on to union.
According to MSTS functional scores, all patients who went on to union had good functional results. Eight patient (32%) developed local recurrence or metastasis, and ultimately
six died of their disease. Two of the paediatric patients in the series went on to develop
significant leg-length discrepancies, both of which had successful limb-lengthening procedures. On the basis of these results, including lower infection and non-union rates, the
authors recommended vascularized fibular autografts as the reconstruction of choice for
long segmental bone defects after tumour resection.[11]

Allograft–Autograft Combination

In order to combine the mechanical advantages of massive allograft with the biological
advantages of a vascularized fibula autograft, Capanna and colleagues described a technique of reconstruction that utilizes both a large structural allograft in conjunction with a
vascularized fibula.[9] Moran and colleagues from the Mayo Clinic reported on a series of
seven paediatric and adolescent patients with extremity sarcoma who were treated with
limb salvage using this reconstructive technique (Figs. 3.3–3.5) The mean follow-up time
was 36 months. All seven patients retained their limb at final follow-up. Fibular autograft
healing occurred by an average of 4 months, while allograft-host healing tended to take
longer, and averaged 9 months. Two cases required secondary bone grafting procedures to
obtain union at the allograft-host junction. There were no infections noted during the study
period. Two patients developed allograft fractures over 2 years after primary surgery. Both
fractures were successfully treated with internal fixation (one also had bone grafting at the
time of fracture repair). Four patients had significant limb-length discrepancies - two
patients with discrepancies less than 2.5 cm were treated with shoe lifts, while two patients
with larger discrepancies were treated with contralateral epiphysiodesis and limb shortening procedures. According to the modified Mankin functional classification, there were
four excellent results and three good results. These results led the authors to conclude that
the Capanna technique is a reliable reconstructive option, and is especially well-suited for
the younger patient, whose higher activity demands and longer life span make allograft
fracture and infection a more likely issue.[33]

Cañadell and San-Julian have described an innovative technique that can improve the
achievement of a safe surgical margin while helping to preserve the native joint surface
in certain appropriately selected children.[8] This technique will be explained in detail in
next chapters.

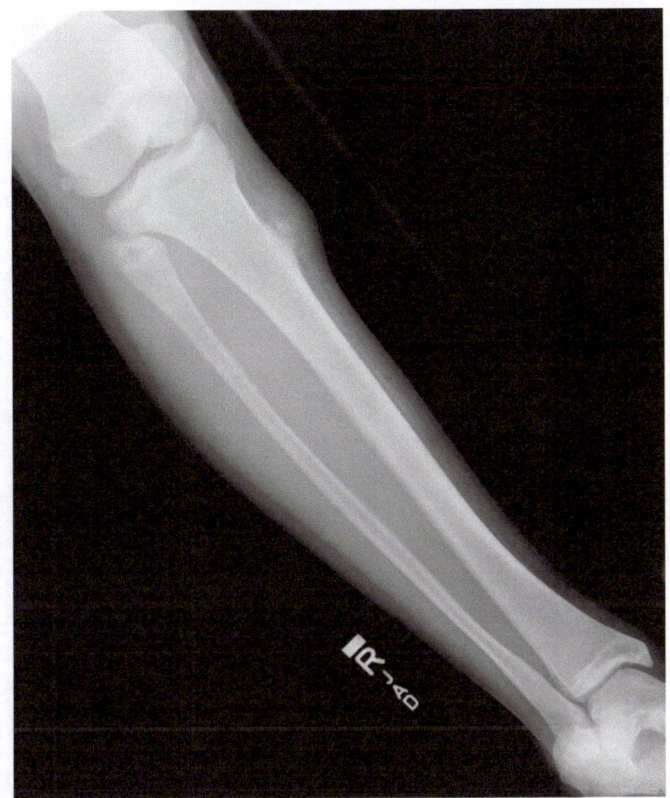

Fig. 3.3 AP x-ray of the tibia, showing a lytic lesion in the proximal tibia of a 14-year-old female with soft tissue extension. Biopsy showed osteosarcoma

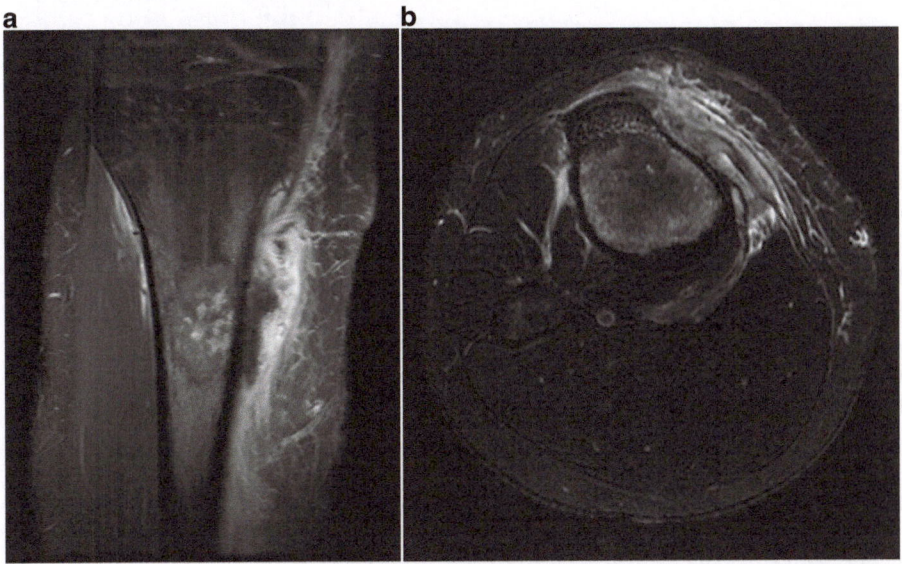

Fig. 3.4 Coronal (**a**) and axial (**b**) MRI images of the patient in Fig. 3.3 following biopsy, showing medullary involvement and soft tissue extension

Fig. 3.5 Lateral x-ray of the patient in Figs. 3.3 and 3.4, following resection through the epiphysis sparing the articular surface. Reconstruction was carried out with an intercalary allograft and intra-medullary vascularized fibular graft. A locking plate was utilized for fixation

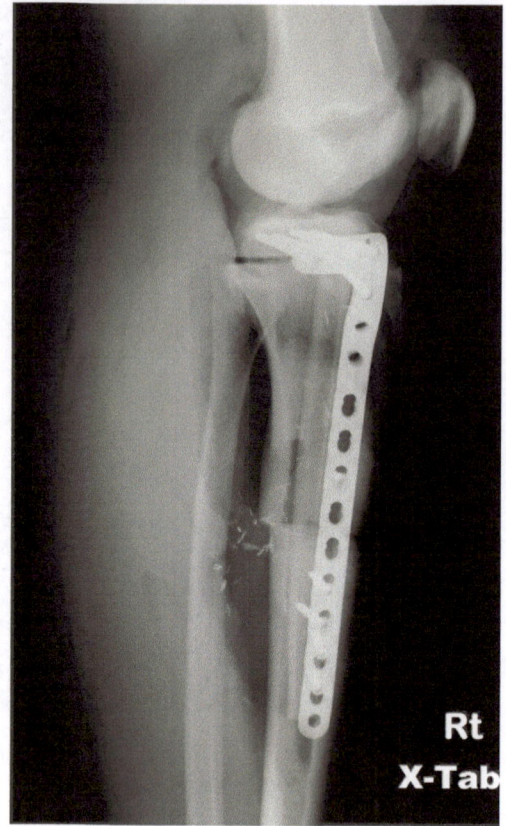

Prosthetic Reconstruction

Non-biological reconstruction after resection of an extremity sarcoma involves placement of a prosthesis to replace the resected bone. The advantages of this technique include better initial fixation which can allow earlier weight-bearing, more predictable function, and lower risk of early complications.[1] Current implants incorporate a modular design, which allows the prosthesis to be assembled to match the defect created at the time of surgery. Additionally, a variety of stem lengths and diameters allow for greater intra-operative flexibility, with cemented and uncemented designs available. Prosthetic designs exist to replace the proximal humerus, proximal femur, distal femur, entire femur, and proximal tibia.

Standard Prostheses

In older children, who are nearing the end of their skeletal growth, a standard, static, adult-type endoprosthesis can be employed, if the expected leg-length discrepancy will be less than 2–3 cm.[1] Additionally, in tumours that occur about the knee, some growth can still be obtained from the remaining physis (i.e. the proximal tibia in distal femur tumours, and vice versa), by placing an uncemented component through a central hole in the physis that would allow the prosthetic stem to slide as the bone continues to grow around it. The distal femoral or proximal tibial physis can then continue to grow without angular deformity, but at a slower rate. The proximal tibia can achieve approximately 80% of normal growth compared to the contralateral leg, whereas the distal femur can achieve about 60%.[1,17]

Standard non-expandable endoprostheses have been used for several decades in adult patients, and have also been utilized in paediatric patients who are nearing skeletal maturity. They have a very good overall track record. In a review of 25 patients (adult and paediatric) treated with a proximal femoral endoprosthetic hemiarthroplasty, the 10-year prosthesis survival rate was 86%. There was one deep infection that was successfully treated with irrigation and debridement and retention of the components; one prosthetic dislocation; and one local recurrence. Three patients had significant acetabular wear, and were planning to undergo acetabular replacement. In each case, the abductor tendons were affixed to the prosthetic trochanter. Some degree of Trendelenburg limp was present in 92% of patients (mild, 56%; moderate 16%; and severe, 20%). Functional outcome was excellent or good in 68%, fair in 28%, and poor in 4%.[13]

Expandable Prostheses

Early endoprostheses were static devices that did not allow for lengthening or growth through the device itself. In order to minimize significant limb-length discrepancies in younger patients, subsequent procedures were often required to either lengthen the ipsilateral extremity (i.e. distraction osteogenesis) or slow the growth of or even shorten the contralateral extremity (i.e. epiphysiodesis, shortening osteotomy). In the 1970s and 1980s, endoprosthetic devices began to incorporate designs that would allow lengthening of the prosthesis itself to allow the affected limb to keep pace with the contralateral limb. The first advance that allowed lengthening was the introduction of modularity. A modular prosthesis could be lengthened by exchanging a mid-body segment of the prosthesis for a longer segment, without the need to revise the entire prosthesis. However, this expansion would require a sizable operative exposure, with excision of the pseudo-capsule that forms around the prosthesis, in order to perform this type of exchange lengthening. Complications including neurovascular injury, joint stiffness, and infection were not uncommon with these procedures.[14]

Later expandable prostheses incorporated designs that would allow for less invasive lengthening procedures over time. These designs worked via one of several mechanisms to allow lengthening, including exchangeable C-collars, ball-bearings, or worm drives. With several of these newer prostheses, expansion procedures could be performed in a percutaneous fashion through a stab incision under fluoroscopic guidance, whereby a screwdriver could be inserted into the lengthening mechanism to expand the prosthesis.[1,4,6,14,17,37]

In 2000, Eckardt and colleagues published a series of 32 endoprostheses that were implanted following malignant bone resection, which could be lengthened by exchanging modular mid-body segments. Over the 12 years that encompassed the study period, four different prosthesis designs were employed. At the time of publication, half of the patients had undergone at least one lengthening exchange procedure. In the 16 patients that had at least 1 lengthening procedure, a total of 32 lengthening procedures were performed. Eighteen of the original 32 patients had a total of 27 complications. These complications included aseptic loosening (five patients), temporary nerve palsy (four patients), prosthesis collapse or mechanical failure (six patients), and local recurrence (two patients). There were no infections noted. Three patients required an operative intervention for knee flexion contractures.[14]

Proximal tibia replacements are often associated with even higher rates of complications, most often due to problems with wound breakdown and infection, and due to the challenges in restoring the extensor mechanism. The group from Birmingham, England reported on a series of expandable proximal tibial prostheses in 20 patients in 2000. Five patients died of their disease, and four others underwent above-knee amputation for complications (two for local recurrence and two for infection). There were seven infections, of which five seemed directly related to open lengthening procedures. The authors determined the risk of infection to be 5.1% per lengthening procedure, and at 10 years, the overall risk of infection was 68%. The patients in the study underwent an average of ten operations, from initial biopsy and prosthesis implant to lengthenings and procedures to address complications (i.e. knee and ankle manipulations, contracture releases, and periprosthetic fractures). However, at final analysis, the average MSTS score was 83%, and the mean leg-length discrepancy was 10 mm. Most patients had a mild-to-moderate extensor lag, as well as some limitation in knee flexion, which is not dissimilar from the results found in proximal tibial endoprosthetic reconstruction in adults.[17]

Even with the development of percutaneous lengthening techniques, patients still required anaesthesia, and the multiple operative procedures increased the risk of infection. In order to obviate the need for repeated surgical procedures, the newest expandable endoprosthetic models have incorporated non-invasive lengthening mechanisms.[1,5,19,37] The most common non-invasive lengthening method utilizes external electromagnetic energy to allow the release of potential energy stored within a spring inside the prosthesis, which allows for expansion.[37] Lengthening can be performed on an outpatient basis, without anaesthesia or an incision required. Generally, the prosthesis is lengthened between 6 and 10 mm per expansion (Figs. 3.6 and 3.7).

Neel and colleagues reported on their experience with this type of prosthesis in 2003. Eighteen prostheses were implanted in 15 patients. Three patients in the study had to have their prosthesis revised to a new expandable prosthesis due to failure of the electromagnetic expansion portion failed. One patient underwent an above-knee amputation 10 months after surgery for an arterial thrombosis. There were eight revisions in seven patients, mostly due to either prosthesis failure or fracture. A total of 60 lengthenings have been performed, with all but two performed on an outpatient basis, and with an average of 8.5 mm of length gained at each procedure. There were no neurovascular injuries or significant loss of range of motion after any lengthening procedure. There were no deep infections. The average MSTS functional score at final follow-up in surviving patients was 90%. All three of the patients that had achieved skeletal maturity by the time of publication had leg-length discrepancies of less than 10 mm.[37]

In 2006, Gupta and colleagues published their experience with a similar non-invasive expandable prosthesis. However, as opposed to a spring, this prosthesis had a magnet, a gearbox, and a telescoping screw. When the magnet was activated by an external

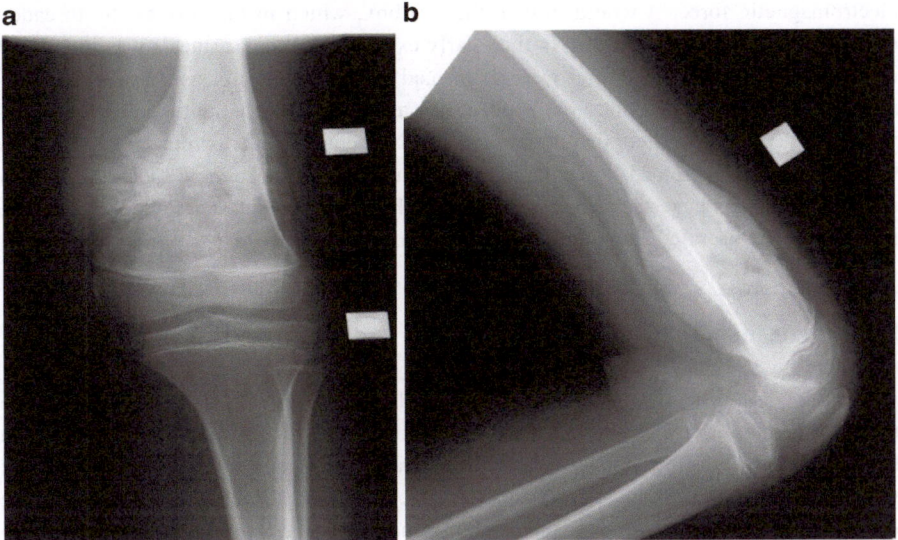

Fig. 3.6 AP (**a**) and lateral (**b**) x-rays of the distal femur, showing Ewing's sarcoma in this 8-year-old patient. Note the large soft tissue mass

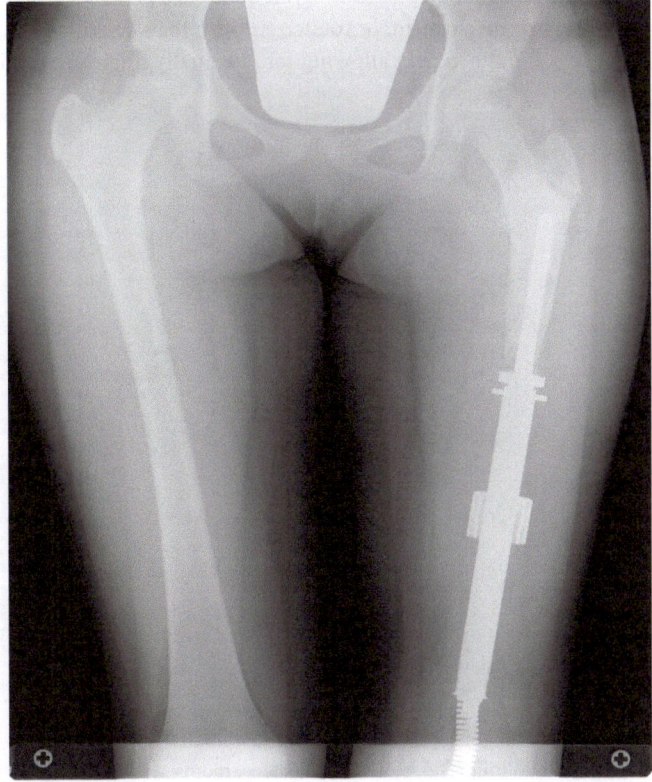

Fig. 3.7 AP scanogram x-ray of the patient in Fig. 3.6, after resection of the distal femur and reconstruction with a epiphysis non-invasive expandable prosthesis

electromagnetic force, it would initiate the gearbox, which in turn drives the threaded screw to lengthen the prosthesis. In their early experience, this prosthesis was implanted into seven patients. Lengthenings were performed on an outpatient basis without anaesthesia. The average length gained per procedure was 4 mm, with patients undergoing anywhere between 1 and 14 lengthening procedures. No neurovascular compromise was seen. One patient developed a 25° knee flexion contracture, which was treated successfully with manipulation under anaesthesia and serial casting. There were no instances of deep infection, implant failure, aseptic loosening, or local tumour recurrence.[19]

Biologic-Prosthetic Combinations

In order to combine some of the advantages of biological and prosthetic reconstruction, the technique of allograft prosthetic composite (APC) reconstruction was devised (Figs. 3.8–3.11). This technique utilizes bulk allograft to replace the missing bone, combined with more standard arthroplasty implants to replace the joint surface. This allows for more options, especially with regards to joint stability and constraint. By resurfacing the joint, the potential for cartilage degradation and joint degeneration 5–10 years after implantation is eliminated.[12] Another advantage of this technique, especially in the proximal femur, proximal tibia, and proximal humerus, is the presence of allograft soft tissue tendon that is still attached at its insertion on the allograft bone. The patient's remaining native hip abductors, knee extensor mechanism, or rotator cuff can than be reconstructed via more reliable soft tissue to soft tissue repair, allowing for potentially improved stability and function.[21]

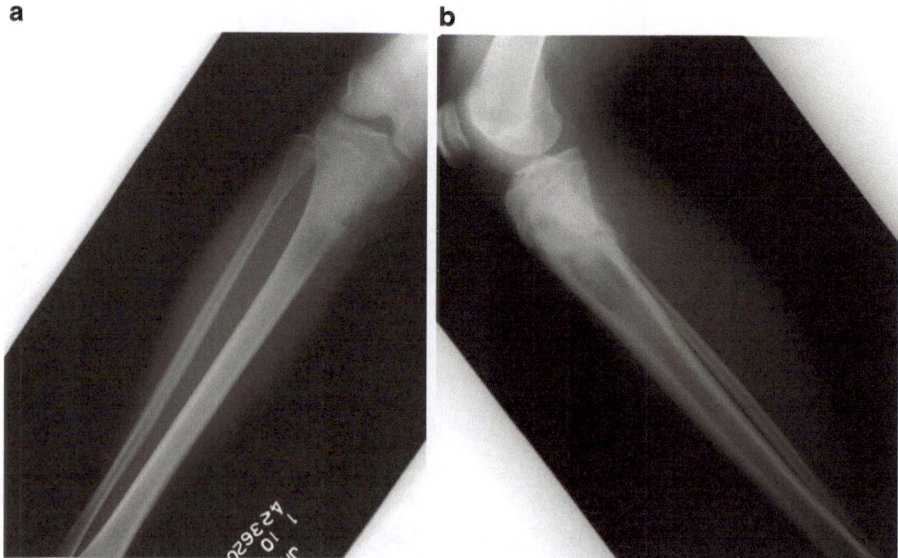

a   b

Fig. 3.8 AP (**a**) and lateral (**b**) x-rays of the tibia demonstrating a mixed lytic and sclerotic lesion in the proximal tibia. Biopsy revealed osteosarcoma

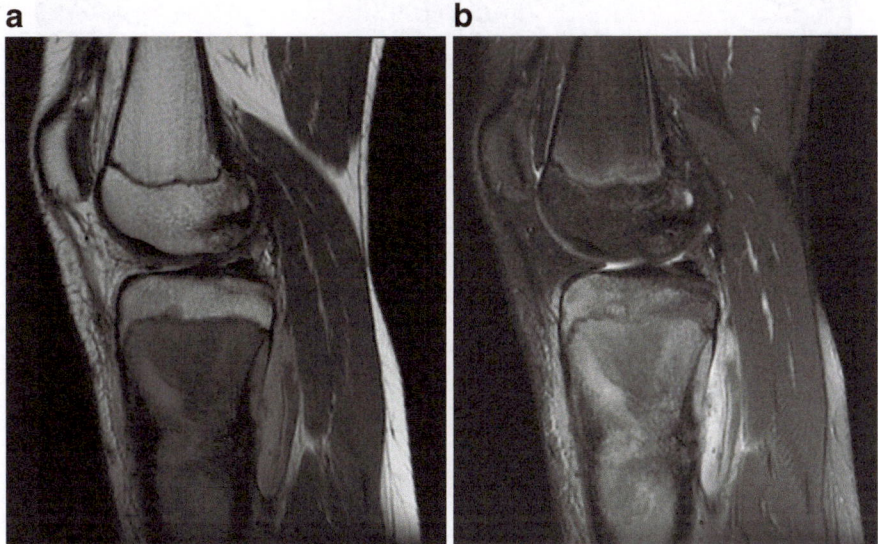

Fig. 3.9 T$_1$- (**a**) and T$_2$- (**b**) weighted sagittal MRI images of the patient in Fig. 3.8, showing the lesion extending to the physis

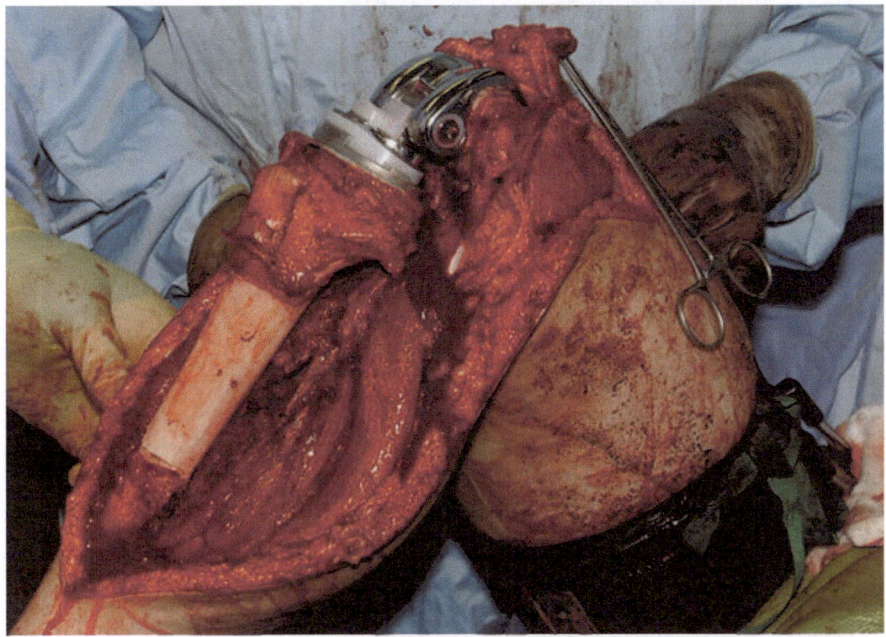

Fig. 3.10 Intra-operative photograph of the patient in Figs. 3.8 and 3.9, showing reconstruction with allograft prosthetic composite

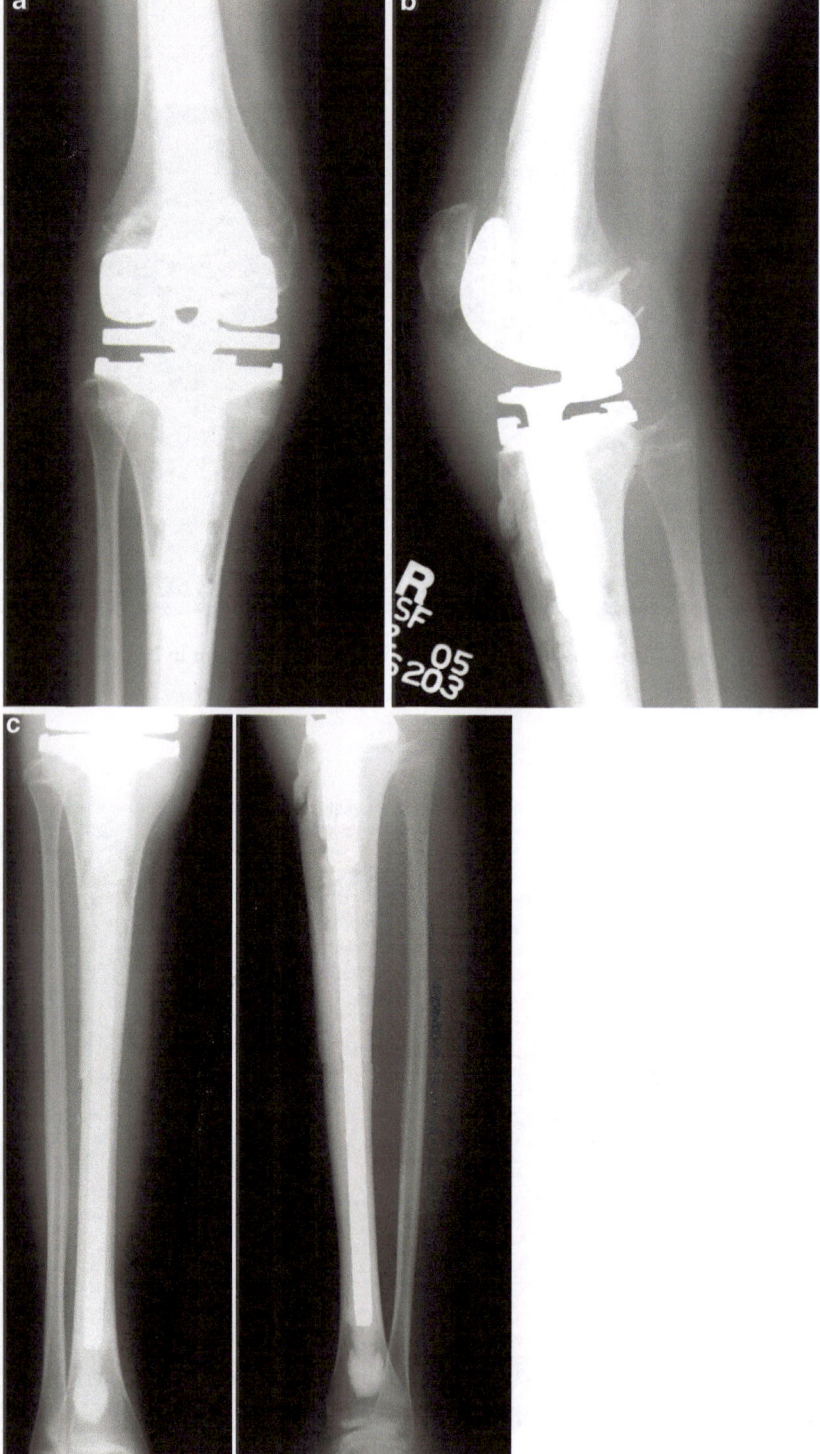

Fig. 3.11 AP (**a**) and lateral (**b**) x-rays of the knee, and AP and lateral x-rays of the tibia (**c**) from the patient in Fig. 3.8, following allograft prosthetic reconstruction

The APC technique can be utilized in the proximal humerus, proximal or distal femur, or proximal tibia. In general, the long stem of the selected prosthetic component is cemented into the allograft, and then ideally press-fit into the remaining host bone. Cement is utilized in the allograft in order to achieve immediate stability as well as longer term stability (since bony ingrowth from the avascular allograft is unlikely), and to minimize the risk of fracturing the allograft from over-stuffing it to obtain a stable press-fit.[21] Press-fit fixation in the host bone can minimize the risk of aseptic loosening.

In a review of 22 patients who underwent APC reconstruction after tumour resection, with an average follow-up of 45.1 months, Hejna and Gitelis found an overall survival rate of 73%, and an average MSTS functional score of 94.3%. There were five allograft–host junction non-unions, four of which healed after subsequent bone grafting procedures.[12,21]

Modified Amputations

In some instances, complete limb salvage may not be feasible for a particular patient. This may be due to very large predicted limb-length discrepancies that would require multiple procedures to correct, difficulty in obtaining size-matched implants or allografts, or social issues that potentially preclude the frequent and long-term follow-up required after limb salvage reconstruction. If an amputation is chosen for definitive treatment, then the level of amputation chosen should be as distal as possible while still ensuring local control of the tumour. Often, this would require a hip disarticulation or high above-knee amputation. However, the ability to preserve a longer residual limb facilitates external prosthetic fitting, which in turn enhances patient function. As such, several types of modified amputation procedures have been described to retain as much residual limb as possible. These include the Van Nes rotationplasty, the tibia turnplasty, and the tibia-hindfoot osteomusculocutaneous rotationplasty.[7,12,39,43]

Van Nes Rotationplasty

Of the three modified amputation techniques listed, the Van Nes rotationplasty leaves the longest residual stump, provides an effective "knee joint," and is a viable alternative to above-knee amputations in selected patients.[7] It was first performed in 1930 by Borggreve for a patient with tuberculosis of the hip; it was later performed in 1932 by Demel and Gold and in 1950 by Van Nes for congenital femoral deficiencies.[15,26,27] The procedure has been employed in the treatment of malignant tumours of the femur since the 1970s.[7,22] In order to perform a successful Van Nes rotationplasty, the sciatic nerve must be preserved; the vascular supply to the lower leg must be salvaged or reconstructed. The tumour is widely excised, leaving the distal lower leg attached by its neurovascular supply. The remaining tibia, with the attached foot, is then rotated 180° and transposed to the remaining distal femur. Tibiofemoral osteosynthesis is achieved using internal fixation devices (Figs. 3.12–3.16). The foot now faces posteriorly, with the remaining, functional ankle joint serving to replace the knee, with the foot acting as a below-knee amputation level stump.[7,22,26,43]

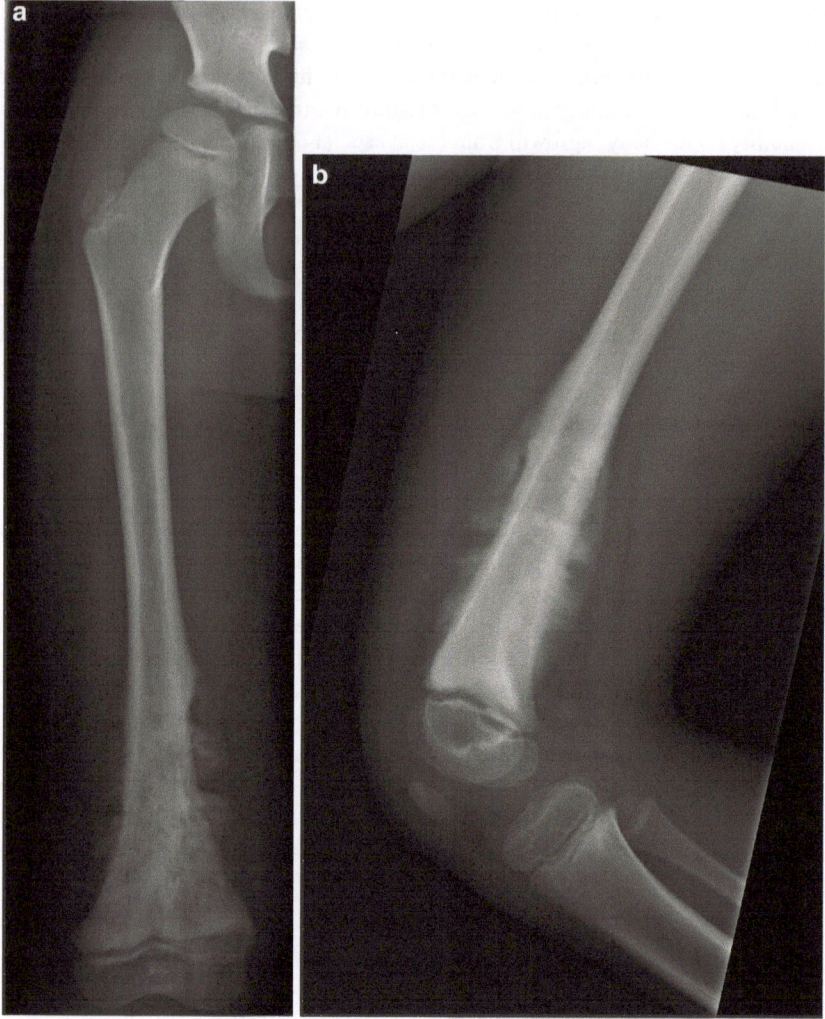

Fig. 3.12 AP x-ray of the femur (**a**) and lateral x-ray of the distal femur (**b**), showing osteosarcoma in a 7-year-old boy

In a study of 12 patients that underwent rotationplasty following resection of a malignant tumour, Cammisa and colleagues reported that functional scores for the rotationplasty patients were statistically equal to those patients that underwent endoprosthetic reconstruction, and statistically better than those patients that underwent above-knee amputation. Disease-free survival was similar for all three groups. One patient had a non-union at the tibiofemoral junction, which was successfully treated with an intra-medullary nail and bone grafting. There were three infections (two superficial and one deep). All complications resolved after treatment, with no functional or long-term consequences. The authors therefore felt that Van Nes rotationplasty was an attractive option for reconstruction after tumour resection, and that it was superior to above-knee amputation.[7]

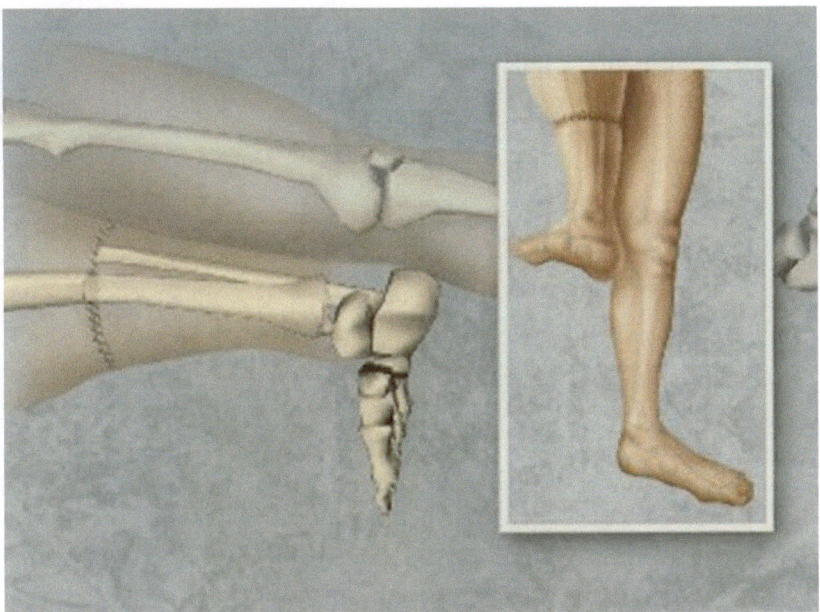

Fig. 3.13 An illustration of rotationplasty. The tibia is rotated 180° and fused to the femur

Hillmann and colleagues published a report comparing endoprosthetic replacement to rotationplasty in 67 patients, both adults and children, with malignant tumours of the distal femur or proximal tibia. Endoprosthetic replacement was performed in 34 patients and rotationplasty in 33. There was no statistically significant difference in the mean MSTS functional score between the two groups (rotationplasty 24; endoprosthesis 25; $p = 0.47$). Fewer patients in the rotationplasty required gait aids for walking long distances. Subjective quality of life scores were significantly higher in the rotationplasty group, and daily activity restriction secondary to pain was significantly lower in the rotationplasty group. The authors did note that cosmetic appearance is likely the biggest drawback concerning rotationplasty.[22] However, several authors feel that the durability and functional advantage of rotationplasty justify the bizarre appearance.[15,22] Others reported that patients were not as bothered by the appearance, and that they considered the procedure to be limb sparing (as opposed to an amputation) since the foot was retained. These patients felt that improved function and mobility more than outweighed the appearance.[25,27]

In an excellent review of rotationplasty published in 1997, Kotz reviewed his experience in 40 patients for whom he performed this procedure. Thirty of the patients were followed for at least 3 years. There were no local recurrences; six patients died of metastatic disease. All patients were ambulating without gait aids, and most reported being able to participate in sports activities. Utilizing the MSTS functional scoring system, the results were excellent in 68%, good in 28.5%, and fair in 3.5%; there were no poor results. Postoperative complications included four patients with vascular thrombosis (three were able to be revascularized and one had to undergo amputation after failure to recanalize the vessels). There were two cases of pseudo-arthrosis at the tibiofemoral junction, both

Fig. 3.14 Intra-operative
photograph during
rotationplasty procedure. The
foot has been rotated 180°. A
plate is utilized for fixation of
the tibia and femur

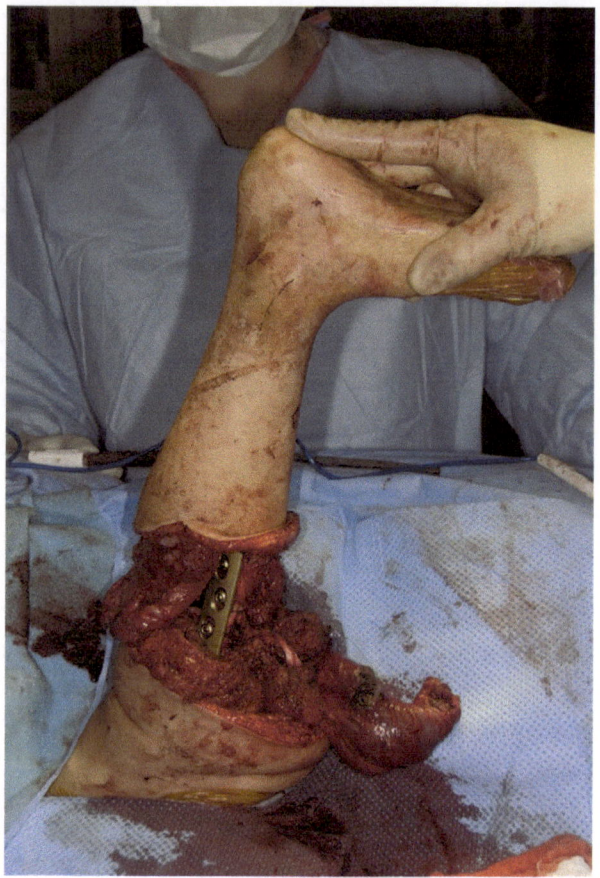

successfully treated with bone grafting and revision internal fixation. There were two cases
of sciatic paresis, one of which resolved spontaneously. Kotz concluded that, although the
indications for rotationplasty were decreasing with advances in extendable endoprostheses
for children, there was still a role for rotationplasty in specific instances, for instance,
proximal tibia tumours for which an amputation would require a below-knee amputation
with a very short stump, or in tumours located more proximally in the femur. There is also
still a role for rotationplasty in developing countries, where endoprostheses are often
unobtainable, and where the infection rate after arthroplasty is unacceptably high.[26]

In their review of limb salvage surgery for skeletally immature patients, Finn and Simon
concluded that rotationplasty offers no compromise of oncological outcome compared to
above-knee amputation. While the complication rate after rotationplasty is higher than that for
amputation, it compares favourably to the rates for other forms of limb salvage. Additionally,
objective data shows that function is significantly improved over above-knee amputation.[15]

When considering someone for rotationplasty, patient selection and pre-operative edu-
cation are critical. The procedure must not compromise the oncological margins, and the
sciatic nerve must be preserved in order for the foot to function as a surrogate knee.

Fig. 3.15 AP radiograph of the right lower extremity showing osteosynthesis of the femur and tibia

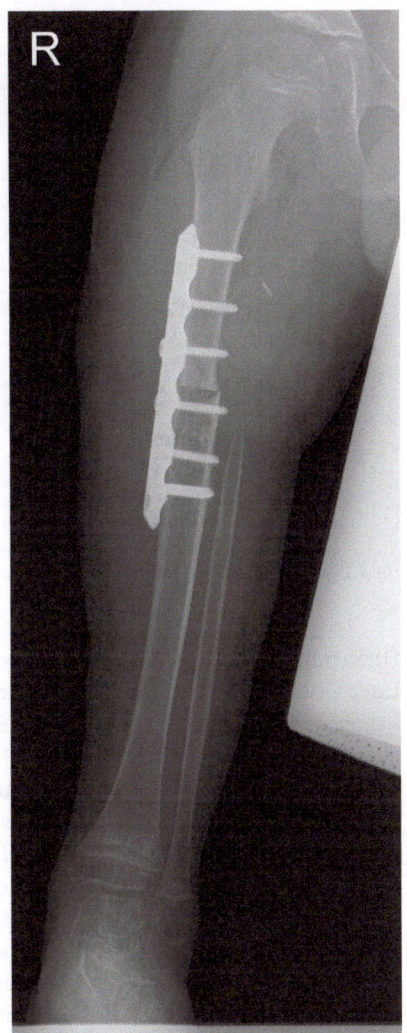

The blood supply to the lower leg and foot must be able to be preserved or reconstructed. Additionally, it is important to educate patients beforehand regarding the anticipated function and physical appearance of the residual limb. It can help to have patients and families view photos or videos that demonstrate the results of rotationplasty, or to even be able to meet with or speak to patients who have previously undergone the procedure.[26]

Tibial Turnplasty

The tibia turnplasty, or turn-up procedure, offers another alternative to a high above-knee amputation. It can be used in the management of long distal femoral bone loss, particularly to salvage multiple previous biological or endoprosthetic reconstruction failures or infections.

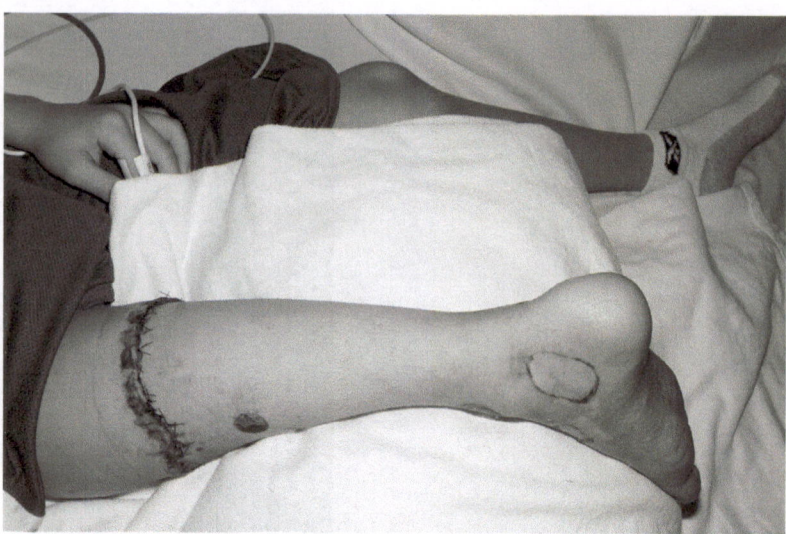

Fig. 3.16 Clinical photograph of rotated foot following wound closure after rotationplasty procedure

Often times, in these patients, such a proximal level for above-knee amputation would not leave a sufficient stump to allow for a functional external prosthesis. Therefore, in order to lengthen the stump and improve prosthetic fitting, remaining tibia can be used as a vascularized autograft. The tibia is rotated 180° on its posterior tibial neurovascular pedicle, such that the distal tibia can be fixed to the remaining femoral stump. In a skeletally immature patient, if the proximal tibial physis can be preserved, then there can be continued longitudinal growth of the stump as well.[31]

McDonald, Scott, and Eckardt reviewed their use of the tibial turn-up procedure in seven patients, three of whom were skeletally immature. Successful osteosynthesis was achieved in all patients, and all were able to ambulate with an above-knee amputation prosthesis. Two patients had post-operative wound complications. One patient ultimately went on to hemipelvectomy subsequent to recurrent tumour. The authors concluded that the tibial turnplasty could be useful to restore femoral stump length in patients who would otherwise require high above-knee amputations, but that it was perhaps best reserved for patients who have had multiple prior surgical failures, deep infections, or those who would be opposed to the appearance of a Van Nes rotationplasty.[31]

Tibia-Hindfoot Osteomusculocutaneous Rotationplasty

In patients with significant tumour involvement or bone loss of the proximal femur, reconstruction options can include endoprosthetic reconstruction, allografts, or allograft–prosthetic composites. In some instances, however, reconstruction may not be possible, for instance, if prior reconstructive efforts have been complicated by repeated deep infections. In these cases, often times a hip disarticulation amputation is required. A hip disarticulation is quite disabling and cosmetically disfiguring, and function with an external prosthesis can be challenging. In order to treat instances such as this, a new procedure was designed that would allow the distal lower extremity to be rotated up as a vascularized autograft on its posterior tibia neurovascular bundle to replace the proximal femur. Skin and soft tissue could be brought up with the bone to fill in any defects as an osteomusculocutaneous flap. The talus and calcaneus are kept with the distal tibia, via their ligamentous attachments. The distal tibia and hindfoot are then rotated 180° in the sagittal plane and 90° in the transverse plane to allow the calcaneal tuberosity to be placed into the acetabulum. The acetabulum is first reamed much like it would be for a hip arthroplasty; the calcaneal tuberosity can be prepared using the reamers that are usually utilized for the femoral head in hip resurfacing procedures. The calcaneal tuberosity is then inserted into the prepared acetabulum, and large screws are placed to facilitate calcaneopelvic fusion. Some "hip joint" motion can then be preserved via the intact tibiotalar and subtalar joints, and the tibia serves as an above-knee amputation stump.[39]

Peterson, Koch, and Wood reported on the performance of this type of rotationplasty (also called a hip-ankle, or Hankle, rotationplasty) in two patients at the Mayo Clinic. Although in their report both patients required this procedure due to extensive loss of the proximal femur and pre-existing deep infection, the procedure could have oncological indications in skeletally immature patients. In the series from Mayo, both patients had successful reconstruction with this technique, and were able to ambulate pain free on standard above-knee amputation prostheses.[39]

Long-Term Outcomes

Many studies have been published reporting on the long-term outcomes in paediatric patients who were treated for extremity sarcomas. Many of these studies compare various techniques with one another. Generally, the oncological and functional results after limb salvage compare favourably to those after amputation.[12,36,44]

In a review published in 2002, Nagarajan and colleagues reported that, while survival is equivalent in limb salvage and amputation procedures, complications tend to be more frequent in the limb salvage group. Additionally, the long-term outcomes with regards to function and quality of life do not appear to be substantially different.[36] However, they noted that limb salvage procedures remain the current practice at most tertiary centres, despite the "higher complication rate, questionable long-term durability, and equivocal improved function and quality of life".[36]

In contrast, Rougraff et al, in a multi-centre study of patients with distal femoral osteosarcoma, reported higher average MSTS functional scores for patients that underwent limb salvage as opposed to those who had amputation. There were no differences between the groups in overall survival or post-operative disease-free periods. There was a higher rate of re-operation in the limb salvage group, but there were no significant differences in the patient's acceptance of the post-operative state, the ability to ambulate, or the amount of pain. There also were no apparent differences in psychosocial outcomes.[40]

Despite the more frequent need for re-operation in limb salvage patients (whether for complications or for limb-lengthening procedures), Wilkins and Miller found that average MSTS functional scores were similar in those limb salvage patients that required at least one subsequent operation compared to those who required no further surgical intervention. In their study of 36 patients with minimum 2-year follow-up, they found that 26 patients needed at least one re-operation (total 54 re-operations performed), while only 10 patients did not need further surgery. There were no significant differences in functional scores in the re-operation group when comparing before and after re-operation, and no differences between the two groups.[45]

Hopyan and colleagues also compared the functional outcomes in paediatric patients who underwent either limb salvage, rotationplasty, or amputation procedures for bone sarcoma. They found that average MSTS functional scores were significantly higher in the limb-sparing group compared to the above-knee amputation group. Additionally, although not statistically significant, the average Toronto Extremity Salvage Scores tended to be higher in the limb-sparing group. They found no significant differences in any psychosocial factors between the three groups.[23]

Another factor for surgeons and patients to consider when choosing between limb salvage and amputation is cost-effectiveness. Grimer and colleagues evaluated the costs associated with endoprosthetic limb salvage and compared that to those associated with amputation, in 1997 prices. They found that, even when adjusting for ongoing limb salvage costs relating to predicted rates of revision surgery (i.e. for aseptic loosening, infection, or implant failure), the overall 20-year cost of amputation is significantly higher. This is likely due to the high cost of sophisticated artificial limbs, the need for regular new prosthesis fabrication, the patient's desire to have a spare prosthesis available, as well as specialized prosthesis for activities such as running or swimming, and others.[18]

Conclusions

Significant multidisciplinary advances have been made in the ways in which we diagnose and treat sarcomas of the extremities. Five-year survival rates have approximately tripled over the last 30 years, but have now seemed to have reached a plateau. Surgical techniques have also advanced considerably over this time period. The great majority of patients with extremity sarcoma are now candidates for limb salvage surgery instead of amputation.

Many different techniques exist to reconstruct a limb after resection of a malignant bone tumour. Each of these techniques has its own advantages and disadvantages. Ultimately, no one procedure will be right for every tumour in every anatomic location in every patient. Each patient must be evaluated on a case-by-case basis. Multiple factors must be considered and prioritized - the patient's life, the extremity, its function, potential leg-length differences, and cosmetic appearance. Additionally, social, socioeconomic, and cultural factors must be accounted for in order to achieve the best outcome for the patient and his or her family.[43] Only when all of these factors are thoroughly evaluated and discussed, can an appropriate treatment plan be devised and embarked upon.

References

1. Abudu A, Grimer R, Tillman R, Carter S. The use of prostheses in skeletally immature patients. *Orthop Clin N Am.* 2006;37:75–84.
2. Alman BA, De Bari A, Krajbich JI. Massive allografts in the treatment of osteosarcoma and Ewing sarcoma in children and adolescents. *J Bone Joint Surg Am.* 1995;77-A:54–64.

3. Arndt CA, Crist WM. Common musculoskeletal tumors of childhood and adolescence. *N Engl J Med.* 1999;341:342–352.
4. Ayoub KS, Fiorenza F, Grimer RJ, Tillman RM, Carter SR. Extensible endoprostheses of the humerus after resection of bone tumors. *J Bone Joint Surg Br.* 1999;81-B:495–500.
5. Baumgart R, Hinterwimmer S, Krammer M, Meunsterer O, Mutschler W. The bioexpandable prosthesis: a new perspective after resection of malignant bone tumors in children. *J Pediatr Hematol Oncol.* 2005;27:452–455.
6. Belthur MV, Grimer RJ, Suneja R, Carter SR, Tillman RM. Extensible endoprostheses for bone tumors of the proximal femur in children. *J Pediatr Orthop.* 2003;23:230–235.
7. Cammisa FP, Glasser DB, Otis JC, Kroll MA, Lane JM, Healey JH. The Van Nes tibial rotationplasty: a functionally viable reconstructive procedure in children who have a tumor of the distal end of the femur. *J Bone Joint Surg Am.* 1990;72-A:1541–1547.
8. Cañadell J, Forriol F, Cara JA, San-Julian M. Removal of metaphyseal bone tumors with preservation of the epiphysis. Physeal distraction before excision In: Cañadell J, San-Julian M, Cara JA, eds. *Surgical Treatment of Malignant Bone Tumors.* Pamplona: Ediciones Universidad de Navarra; 1995:153–160.
9. Capanna R, Bufalini C, Campanacci C. A new technique for reconstruction of large metadiaphyseal bone defects: a combined graft (allograft shell plus vascularized fibula). *Orthop Traumatol.* 1993;2:159–177.
10. Cara JA, Cañadell J. Limb salvage for malignant bone tumors in young children. *J Pediatr Orthop.* 1994;14:112–118.
11. Chen CM, Disa JJ, Lee HY, et al. Reconstruction of extremity long bone defects after sarcoma resection with vascularized fibula flaps: a 10-year review. *Plast Reconstr Surg.* 2007;119:915–924.
12. DiCaprio MR, Friedlaender GE. Malignant bone tumors: limb sparing versus amputation. *J Am Acad Orthop Surg.* 2003;11:25–37.
13. Donati D, Zavatta M, Gozzi E, Giacomini S, Campanacci L, Mercuri M. Modular prosthetic replacement of the proximal femur after resection of a bone tumor: a long-term follow-up. *J Bone Joint Surg Br.* 2001;83-B:1156–1160.
14. Eckardt JJ, Kabo JM, Kelly CM, et al. Expandable endoprosthesis reconstruction in skeletally immature patients with tumors. *Clin Orthop.* 2000;373:51–61.
15. Finn HA, Simon MA. Limb-salvage surgery in the treatment of osteosarcoma in skeletally immature individuals. *Clin Orthop.* 1991;262:108–118.
16. Gonzalez-Herranz P, Burgos-Flores J, Ocete-Guzman JG, et al. The management of limb-length discrepancies in children after treatment of osteosarcoma and Ewing's sarcoma. *J Pediatr Orthop.* 1995;15:561–565.
17. Grimer RJ, Belthur M, Carter SR, Tillman RM, Cool P. Extendible replacements of the proximal tibia for bone tumors. *J Bone Joint Surg Br.* 2000;82-B:255–260.
18. Grimer RJ, Carter SR, Pynsent PB. The cost-effectiveness of limb salvage for bone tumors. *J Bone Joint Surg Br.* 1997;79-B:558–561.
19. Gupta A, Meswania J, Pollock R, et al. Non-invasive distal femoral expandable endoprosthesis for limb-salvage surgery in pediatric tumors. *J Bone Joint Surg Br.* 2006;88-B:649–654.
20. Gurney J, Swensen A, Bulterys M, et al. Malignant bone tumors. In: Ries LA, Smith MA, Gurney JG, eds. Malignant bone tumors. Cancer Statistics Branch, National Cancer Institute, SEER Program; 1999:99–110.
21. Gurney JG, Young JL, Roffers SD, et al. Soft tissue sarcomas. In: Ries LA, Smith Ma, Gurney JG, eds. Soft tissue sarcomas. Cancer Statistics Branch, National Cancer Institute, SEER Program; 1999:11–123.
22. Hejna MJ, Gitelis S. Allograft prosthetic composite replacement for bone tumors. *Sem Surg Onc.* 1997;13:18–24.
23. Hillmann A, Hoffmann C, Gosheger G, Krakau H, Winkelmann W. Malignant tumor of the distal part of the femur of proximal part of the tibia: endoprosthetic replacement or rotationplasty. *J Bone Joint Surg Am.* 1999;81-A:462–468.

24. Hopyan S, Tan JW, Graham HK, Torode IP. Function and upright time following limb salvage, amputation, and rotationplasty for pediatric sarcoma of bone. *J Pediatr Orthop.* 2006;26:405–408.

25. Hosalkar HS, Dormans JP. Limb sparing surgery for pediatric musculoskeletal tumors. *Pediatr Blood Cancer.* 2004;42:295–310.

26. Jacobs PA. Limb salvage and rotationplasty for osteosarcoma in children. *Clin Orthop.* 1984;188:217–222.

27. Kotz R. Rotationplasty. *Sem Surg Oncol.* 1997;13:34–40.

28. Kotz R, Salzer M. Rotation-plasty for childhood osteosarcoma of the distal part of the femur. *J Bone Joint Surg Am.* 1982;64-A:959–969.

29. Kumta SM, Cheng JCY, Li CK, et al. Scope and limitations of limb-sparing surgery in childhood sarcomas. *J Pediatr Orthop.* 2002;22:244–248.

30. LewisVO. Limb salvage in the skeletally immature patient. *Curr Oncol Rep.* 2005;7:285–292.

31. Manoso MW, Boland PJ, Healey JH, Tyler W, Morris CD. Acetabular development after bipolar hemiarthroplasty for osteosarcoma in children. *J Bone Joint Surg Br.* 2005;87-B:1658–1662.

32. McDonald DJ, Scott SM, Eckardt JJ. Tibial turn-up for long distal femoral bone loss. *Clin Orthop.* 2001;383:214–220.

33. Mnaymneh W, Malinin TI, Lackman RD, et al. Massive distal femoral osteoarticular allografts after resection of bone tumors. *Clin Orthop.* 1994;303:103–115.

34. Moran SL, Shin AY, Bishop AT. The use of massive bone allograft with intramedullary free fibula flap for limb salvage in a pediatric and adolescent population. *Plast Reconstr Surg.* 2006;118:413–419.

35. Musculo DL, Ayerza MA, Aponte-Tinao L, Farfalli G. Allograft reconstruction after sarcoma resection in children younger than 10 years old. Clin Orthop. 2008; May 28 e-publication ahead of print.

36. Musculo DL, Ayerza MA, Aponte-Tinao LA, Ranalletta M. Use of distal femoral osteoarticular allografts in limb salvage surgery. *J Bone Joint Surg Am.* 2005;87-A:2449–2455.

37. Nagarajan R, Neglia JP, Clohisy DR, Robison LL. Limb salvage and amputation in survivors or pediatric lower extremity bone tumors: what are the long term implications? *J Clin Oncol.* 2002;20:4493–4501.

38. Neel MD, Wilkins RM, Rao BN, Kelly CM. Early multicenter experience with a noninvasive expandable prosthesis. *Clin Orthop.* 2003;415:72–81.

39. Ortiz-Cruz E, Gebhardt MC, Jennings LC, Springfield DS, Mankin HJ. The results of transplantation of intercalary allografts after resection of tumors. *J Bone Joint Surg Am.* 1997; 79-A:97–106.

40. Peterson CA, Koch LD, Wood MB. Tibia-hindfoot osteomusculocutaneous rotationplasty with calcaneopelvic arthrodesis for extensive loss of bone from the proximal part of the femur: a report of two cases. *J Bone Joint Surg Am.* 1997;79-A:1504–1509.

41. Rougraff BT, Simon MA, Kneisl JS, Greenberg DB, Mankin HJ. Limb salvage compared with amputation for osteosarcoma of the distal end of the femur. *J Bone Joint Surg.* 1994;76-A:649–656.

42. San-Julian M, Dolz R, Garcia-Barrecheguren E, et al. Limb salvage in bone sarcomas in patients younger than age 10. *J Pediatr Orthop.* 2003;23:753–762.

43. Van Kampen M, Grimer RJ, Carter SR, Tillman RM, Abudu A. Replacement of the hip in children with a tumor in the proximal part of the femur. *J Bone Joint Surg Am.* 2008;90-A:785–795.

44. Weisstein JS, Goldsby RE, O'Donnell RJ. Oncologic approaches to pediatric limb preservation. *J Am Acad Orthop Surg.* 2005;13:544–554.

45. Wilkins RM, Miller CM. Reoperation after limb preservation surgery for sarcomas of the knee in children. *Clin Orthop.* 2003;412:153–161.

Location of Sarcomas Within Bone: The Growth Plate

4

Francisco Forriol, Mikel San-Julian, and José Cañadell

Abstract Most malignant bone tumours are located in the metaphysis near a growth plate. On tumoural resection, better functional results are achieved when a nearby joint is preserved. The growth plate could represent a barrier to tumour spread in some cases. Physeal distraction has been reported to be an orthopaedic technique useful in various situations. We now describe a new application for this technique.

Location of Malignant Bone Tumours

Malignant bone tumours represent 5.6% of the total malignant disease in patients under 15 years of age and 0.5% of all human tumours. The most common tumours during childhood and adolescence are osteosarcoma and Ewing's sarcoma. In about 75% of these young patients, the lesions are located near a growth plate. Historically, these tumours were treated by amputation, although this did not increase the survival rate; when surgery was the only method of treatment, the survival rate was less than 20%, and only patients with localised disease had any chance of survival. With the advent of chemotherapy, the management of malignant tumours was much improved. More accurate diagnoses due to advances in imaging technology, improvement in surgical techniques and the use of preoperative chemotherapy have increased the indications for limb salvage.

Limb preservation has particularly been facilitated by preoperative chemotherapy. For example, since 1981 in our department, the use of intra-arterial chemotherapy in the treatment of osteosarcoma[9] has allowed us to increase the indications for limb salvage to almost 100%. Consequently, we have become more and more interested in limb-reconstruction techniques. These procedures require a multidisciplinary approach in which the surgeon is joined by radiologists, pathologists and oncologists. The local recurrence rate with lower limb salvage is now similar to that for above-the-knee amputation,[52] and survival rates are also comparable.[4,37,48,52]

Francisco Forriol (✉)
Research Department, FREMAP, Ctra Pozuelo, 61, Majadahonda, Madrid 28220, Spain
e-mail: fforriol@fremap.es

J. Cañadell and M. San-Julian (eds.), *Pediatric Bone Sarcomas: Epiphysiolysis Before Excision*,   **57**
DOI: 10.1007/978-1-84882-130-9_4, © Springer-Verlag London Limited 2011

4

Functional Results in Articular Versus Diaphyseal Locations

Limb salvage includes two operative procedures. The first is tumour excision, and its adequacy can be judged simply by the rate of local recurrence. To cure primary tumours it is necessary to perform en bloc resection of all macroscopic disease, including the biopsy scar. The degree of osteotomy required to allow a safe margin is determined on the basis of the intramedullary spread of tumour as revealed by imaging methods. There is no complete accordance among orthopaedic surgeons about what constitutes a "safe margin", but most of them consider 5 cm beyond the tumour as sufficient. Articular cartilage is thought to prevent tumour spread in most cases, and therefore can be considered as a safe margin. For this reason, in tumours involving the epiphysis, resection of the joint is adequate.

The second procedure is reconstruction. The selection of a method of reconstruction must consider the effects of any secondary deformity, as predicted by the amount of removed physeal cartilage, on function. We believe that the choice of the type of reconstruction should be based on each patient's age, size, functional demands and desires; the surgeon's experience is also an important factor. A few patients with a primary tumour of the scapula, clavicle, proximal fibula or rib can be treated by simple resection and suffer only minimal functional impairment.

Resections requiring reconstruction can be subdivided into two major categories: diaphyseal resections and articular resections. Intercalary bone grafts are, in our opinion, the correct treatment for diaphyseal resections *when it is possible to preserve the epiphysis*. The functional results with intercalary reconstruction after diaphyseal resection are better than the results after articular resection[39] (Fig. 4.1a, b).

Compared with metallic implants, bone grafts offer many advantages, including tendinous reattachment, incorporation of the graft to the host bone and longevity.[21] The growth plate has traditionally been considered capable of blocking the spread of a tumour, but this barrier is not impenetrable. In limb preserving procedures, preserving the joint near the tumour is important for achieving better functional results. Unfortunately, it is not possible to preserve the epiphysis in all cases.

Articular resections pose the most complex problems of reconstruction in oncological surgery.[50]

Morphology of Growth Cartilage

Physeal growth cartilage is the longitudinal growth organ of the long bones. Rubin refers to it as the *physis*, because it lies between the epiphysis and the metaphysis; its structure is at once elastic enough to permit interstitial growth, and rigid enough to constitute part of the skeleton.

The cells of growth cartilage are the chondrocytes, which direct the whole process of enchondral ossification and are responsible for controlling the extent of growth in the long bones during postnatal development. The mechanical properties of growth cartilage depend on the extracellular matrix which is produced and maintained by the chondrocytes.

Growth cartilage chondrocytes remain in the same relative position throughout their life. Although their two most important states are proliferation and hypertrophy, which includes the mineralisation of the matrix before bone reabsorption during vascular invasion, a physeal

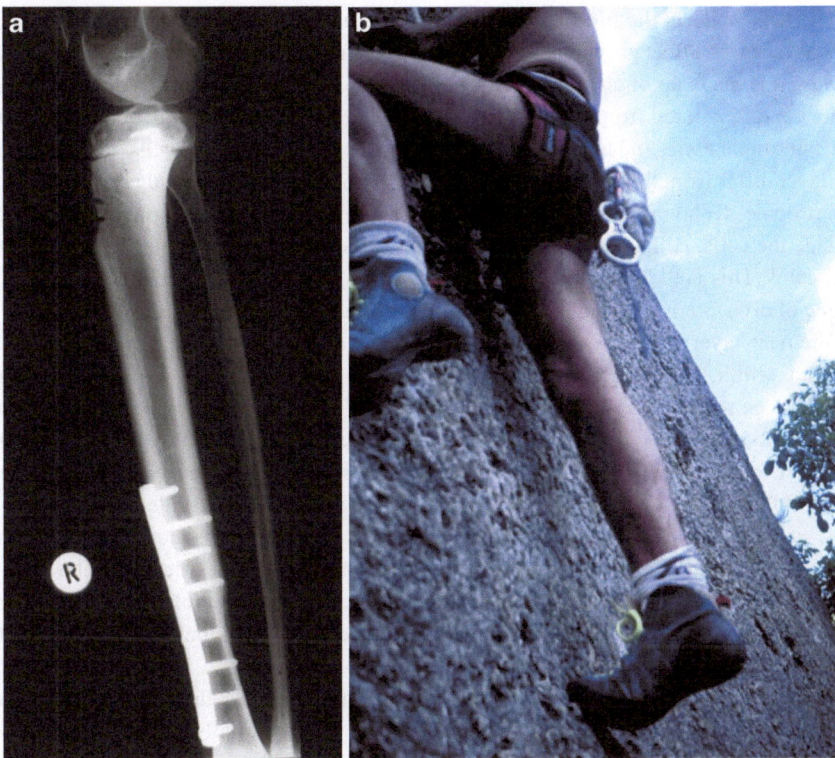

Fig. 4.1 (a) Intercalary reconstruction of the tibia by using an allograft after resection of an osteosarcoma. Note the holes for patellar tendon reattachment. (b) In this case, preservation of the epiphysis allowed the patient to do sporting activities such as climbing

chondrocyte goes through several phases, each of which is characterised by a predominant functional activity. These phases occur synchronically: the youngest chondrocytes are proliferating cells, whilst the oldest are to be found in regions of vascular invasion.

The layers of chondrocytes arranged between the centre of ossification and the bone metaphysis have been well described in terms of both morphology and function. Four different layers can be distinguished: the gemiral zone, the proliferative zone, the hypertrophic zone and the degenerative zone.

However, other authors such as Jee[29] and Quacci et al[44] consider that from the morphological point of view there are six layers: reserve, proliferation, maturation, hypertrophy, degeneration and calcification, which reflect different function. The three layers nearest to the epiphysis are responsible for the proliferation of cartilage cells, while the three closest to the metaphysis are thought to bring about mineralisation of the pericellular matrix.

The layer nearest to the epiphysis, the *reserve, support* or *germinal* layer, seems to be responsible for latitudinal growth. It has a structure which is reminiscent of hyalin cartilage, as its cells are small and round, with an irregular distribution. The predominant collagen is of type II, and the fibres are arranged so as to act as a barrier against the secondary centre of ossification in the epiphysis. This layer produces the matrix and stores nutrients.[47]

The next layer is the proliferative layer, which has vertical chondrogenic activity and does not seem to affect growth in width. An informal name for this layer is "stacks of coins" because it is made up of chondrocytes arranged in columns parallel to the longitudinal axis of the bone, separated from each other by septa. The matrix is a continuation of the matrix of the germinal zone, and has the same biochemical composition. The cells of the proliferative layer differ from those of the germinal/reserve zone in being generally larger, in having hypertrophic Golgi apparatus and in having large outlines of endoplasmic reticulum. Outside the cells, collagen fibrillae surround each chondrocyte, forming a kind of nest for each cell.[18] This is the only zone of the physis in which chondrocytes divide, and the high degree of division means that the cells are flattened and slightly irregular in shape.

The next layers, hypertrophy and degeneration, do not contribute to growth in either length or width. The hypertrophic zone is about 15–17 chondrocytes across and has traditionally been regarded as having two parts: a region of maturation lying above a region of degeneration. There is morphological and biochemical evidence that hypertrophic cells in the lower region are viable, with an active metabolism, and capable of controlling calcification of the matrix. Found in this area is X-type collagen, which is typical of hypertrophic cells, as well as of other macromolecules which make up the matrix, such as the structural protein S-100 and FGF b. The presence of these macromolecules demonstrates that the hypertrophic chondrocytes are highly differentiated cells playing a role in enchondral ossification. When the hypertrophic cells die, they leave a cavity which becomes subject to vascular invasion and is filled by osteogenic cells.

According to Poole et al,[43] growth cartilage is made up of cells from the reserve and proliferation zones which go through a process until they are finally calcified after becoming hypertrophic. Small rounded cells turn into a group of flattened cells in the proliferative zone, which shows that there is a change in the extracellular matrix and in the walls separating one cell group from another.

As described above, the metaphyseal portion of growth cartilage is subject to destruction followed by the formation of bone tissue throughout the remains of the cartilaginous matrix. Calcification results from the penetration by cells and capillary knots of the gaps left by the degenerated chondrocytes.

Metaphyseal capillaries have no basal membrane and possess large pores. Moreover, the endothelial cells are only loosely connected. Consequently, these capillaries are leaky to plasma and blood cell elements.

The osteoblasts which accompany the vessels are arranged in a mononuclear layer on top of the remains of the longitudinal calcified septa, covering them with osteoid tissue and forming primary spongy bone.

Physeal Vascularisation

The three main sources of vascular supply to the metaphysis are[8]: the feeder artery, the arteries penetrating the metaphysis and the arteries between the bone and the perichondrium.

The feeder artery brings blood to the central metaphyseal area and has peripheral branches with small vessels that are distributed along the inside of the spongy bone.

The central longitudinal branches reach the growth cartilage, resulting in a tree-like vascular pattern. A considerable number of metaphyseal vessels deriving from the articular arteries also contribute to the vascular supply of long bone metaphysis and growth cartilage. All these vessels end in vascular knots or clusters of capillaries just beneath the last intact transverse septum at the base of the cartilaginous part of the growth cartilage.[7] The feeder artery contributes up to 80% of the blood which reaches the metaphysis and in particular irrigates the central part of the metaphysis. The more peripheral areas are irrigated by the perichondral-osseous arteries originating in the arteries of the corresponding joint, which form an anastomotic vascular system that reaches the peripheral structures of the growth cartilage, particularly Ranvier's nodule.

The metaphyseal vascular supply to the growth cartilage plays a fundamental role in the progressive formation of enchondral bone. Injury to these vessel, whether consequent to surgery[60] or to a disease such as rickets,[51] results in an increase in the hypertrophic zone and in the cartilaginous matrix.

The epiphysis receives its vascular supply from one or more vessels which penetrate the cartilage and branch out inside it. The epiphyseal vascular supply to growth cartilage is characterised by small arterial branches coming from the intra-epiphyseal arteries, which ramify to irrigate the proliferative layer of growth cartilage. However, arterial branches of the epiphyseal vessels do not extend into the cartilaginous part of the physis,[7] and so the hypertrophic layer of growth cartilage is free of vascularisation.

The two most important circulatory systems, constituted respectively by epiphyseal and metaphyseal vessels, are separated both functionally and morphologically[9] (Fig. 4.2).

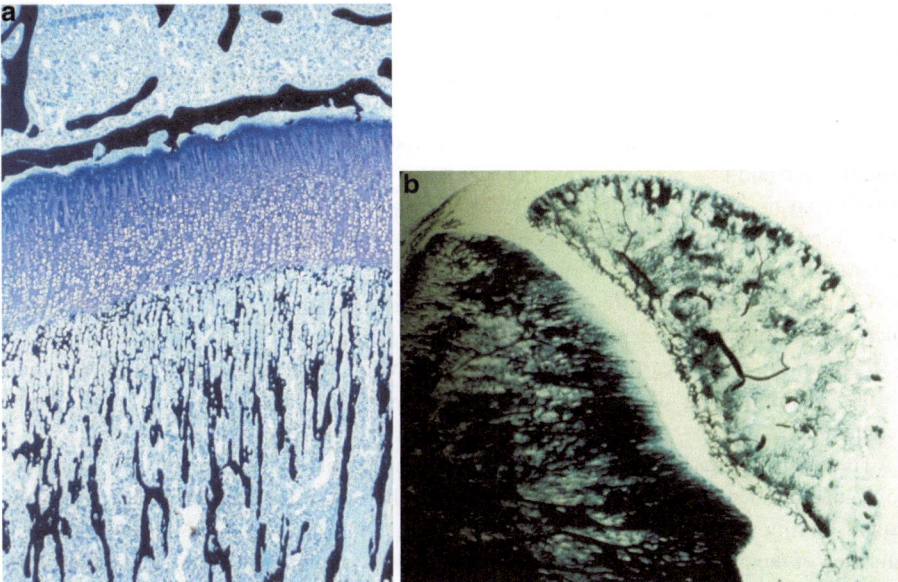

Fig. 4.2 Indian ink injection and spatenholz stain showing no vascular anastomoses between metaphyseal and epiphyseal vessels

There are direct and indirect indications of the function of vascular supply to growing bone. Interruption of vascularisation can lead to necrosis or segmentation of the epiphysis, producing severe deformities.

In this respect, congenital or traumatic arterial and venous fistulae are a common cause of distal overgrowth in bones. Such growth is above all latitudinal, although it may be longitudinal, with an increase in cortical thickness. The influence on immature bone of stasis after a tourniquet has been in position for a long time is an increase in latitudinal growth.[23]

Further, the implantation of various materials in the medullary canal stimulates bone growth, particularly enchondral growth.[31,58,60] Deperiostisation[31,55] and diaphyseal fractures also stimulate growth.

Finally, the suppression of metaphyseal vascularisation produces an increase in the height of the physis.[13,61] Trueta[60] concluded that in less fertile cartilage there is less epiphyseal vascularisation, a greater number of columns irrigated by the same vessel, and a greater distance between the terminal vessels and the proliferating cells.

Experiments on Growth Cartilage: Experimental Physeal Distraction

During growth, the area next to the physis is an ideal focus for lengthening methods because of its special features with regard to bone healing.[7,24,27,28,32,46,64] Traction of growth cartilage produces a fracture which makes it possible to lengthen the bone in a single surgical operation and achieve rapid consolidation without need for section of the skin or osteotomy.

In children, lesions of growth cartilage are frequent. Injury in traction is uncommon as accidents tend to involve sliding strains which, because the physes usually have an uneven, undulate, surface, act uniformly and simultaneously on the whole of the growth cartilage. In the case of many bone types, epiphyseal plates form, in some individuals, the greatest possible angle with the corresponding planes of shear strain.

The distal epiphysis of the femur in the lamb, like that of man, has four bony mamelons, two anterior and two posterior, two inner and two outer, which penetrate four cavities in the metaphysis. The space between the two surfaces if filled by the growth cartilage, which, seen from the front, has a "V" shape. This arrangement prevents separation caused by shear strains.

Changes in tension in different areas of the periosteum may be a factor which leads to increased growth in certain parts of the physis.[30] In injuries which only affect the metaphyseal part of the growth cartilage, this increased growth may be a temporary process which results in broadening of the physis. Good metaphyseal vascularisation ensures rapid regeneration.

The epiphyseal part of the physis comprising the germinal layer is much more sensitive to trauma because such trauma not only disturbs the functional balance of the physis but can also bring about destruction of growth cartilage. The ensuing rapid process of mineralisation of the physis may mean that the physis becomes partly or completely joined onto the primary centre of ossification, and that a bony bridge be formed between the epiphysis and the metaphysis. This may be due to necrosis in the growth cartilage caused by compression or by damage to the blood supply.

The prognosis after a partial delay of growth depends on age and sex. The closure of the physis takes place earlier in females than males. The site of the lesion is another important factor as not all physes contribute in the same way to bone growth; neither do all physes close at the same time. The displacement of the lesion also affects the prognosis: the greater the displacement, the greater the likelihood of damage affecting growth. Complete closure of the physis in conjunction with total degeneration of the growth cartilage is very unusual and brings growth to a complete halt.

Epiphyseal detachment is not usually the result of a direct mechanism; most detachments are caused indirectly, by forced varus or valgus combined with hyperextension. The insertions of muscles and ligaments play an important part in this mechanism.

Pietravissa[42] studied the pathogeny of epiphyseal detachments in cadavers and in animals under anaesthetic by stripping long bones of their musculature and then subjecting these bones to axial, varus and valgus traction, hyperextension and articular hyperflexion and tension associated with abnormal movements. Harris[22] developed a simple experimental model to produce tibial epiphyseal detachment by crossing the epiphysis with a pin joined to a bucket into which he gradually added sand until the break occurred. Bright and Elmore[6] repeated this in rats, and for cartilage. They transfixed both sides of the physis, applied a force of axial traction or traction with a rotational element, and then studied the break line in connection with the force applied. Oliete,[38] after an experimental study with rabbits, concluded that the most important conditioning factors were the animal's age and sex, the site of the epiphysis, and the point at which the force was applied. He demonstrated that the most fragile cartilages are those which have the simplest physeal architecture.

Skak et al[53] found no differences between the sexes in their review article on epiphysiolysis, which has often been considered to be commoner in males than females in the ratio 6:1. This ratio has been explained by the greater aggression of boys at play. However, the force necessary to produce epiphysiolysis increases greatly when oestrogens are given.[22] Various studies corroborate this statement. In rat *tibiae* the resistance of the growth cartilage is greater in females than in males of the same age.[6] Oliete[38] also concluded that female rabbits had more resistant growth cartilage, a lower frequency of epiphysiolysis, and that epiphysiolysis was simpler in the wrist and distal humerus.

In contrast to these in vitro studies, we concur with Weber et al[63] and Rang[45] in believing that the capsular insertions and articular support ligaments protect the physis.

The incidence of physeal lesions peaks in puberty, when their effect on growth is minimal. However, the disadvantage of lesions at this age is that they will only rarely correct spontaneously: the potential for spontaneous corrections falls with age after 10–12 years. Approximately 10% of paediatric fractures cause injury to the epiphyseal region, and growth may be impaired in 10% of damaged epiphyses.

Fjeld et al[20] established that daily distraction of 0.25% of bone length, over a period of between 5 and 9 days, brings about epiphyseal separations in animal models. In all experimental studies on physeal distraction, separation of the growth cartilage from the metaphysis has been observed.[12,28,36,46] When forces are applied in traction, epiphysiolysis of type I according to Salter and Harris's classification[49] is always achieved.

When diaphyseo-epiphyseal distraction is performed in a growing bone, breakage occurs in the zone of least resistance, that is, the physis (Fig. 4.3).

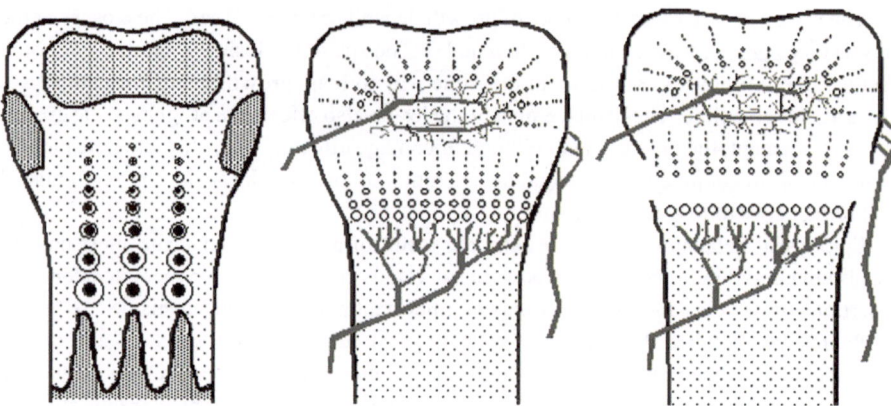

Fig. 4.3 Diagram showing the rupture in the metaphyseal part of a growth plate on application of the physeal distraction technique

At first, the cartilaginous tissue suffers a deformation. However, if bone lengthening is the goal, the metaphysis must be separated from the epiphysis to produce epiphysiolysis[27,41] and the consequent bone neoformation in the area of lengthening.[24,33–35] In the course of this process, the periosteum breaks where the perichondral ring has been inserted. This break produces a haematoma which fills the gap[19,27] and which is later replaced by fibrous tissue.[33–35] Newly formed bone deposition proceeds from the intact periosteum as well as from the epiphyseal and metaphyseal portions[33–35,46,57] of the bone. The characteristic pattern of grooves in the lengthening area, which can be seen by radiology, reflects the mineralisation of the collagen fibres which are arranged lengthways. Occasionally, a radiolucid area can be observed in the lengthening area.[33–35]

De Pablos and Cañadell[16,17] demonstrated that, irrespective of the daily distraction rate, epiphysiolysis is always produced. Their research established a relationship between the morphological variations in the growth cartilage and the rate of distraction used. In sheep *femora* subject to lengthening at 0.5 mm/day, the cartilage remained normal throughout (Fig. 4.4). However, *femora* lengthened by 1 mm/day, and particularly those lengthened by 2 mm/day, were found to have obvious injuries 45 days and 4 months later.

According to some authors,[1,2,6,14] a gradual distraction force of low intensity acting symmetrically on the growth plate can bring about bone growth without producing epiphysiolysis. This constitutes what the Verona School call *chondrodiastasis*. Along these lines, Sledge and Noble[54] found that stimulation of the growth cartilage by applying distractional forces of 1–2 kg on the distal femoral physis in rabbits resulted in hyperplasia of the physis, with an increase in cell mitosis and a rise in polysaccharide sulphate synthesis.

Spriggins et al[56] used fixators equipped with instrumentation to study the forces of physeal distraction in rabbits. They detected two patterns of behaviour. In one group the forces increased to maximum values of 20–32 N, and then decreased until the next distraction. This indicated breakage of the growth cartilage, with the associated hyperplasia. In the other group, forces with lower values, 6–18 N, were reached at the end of the distraction

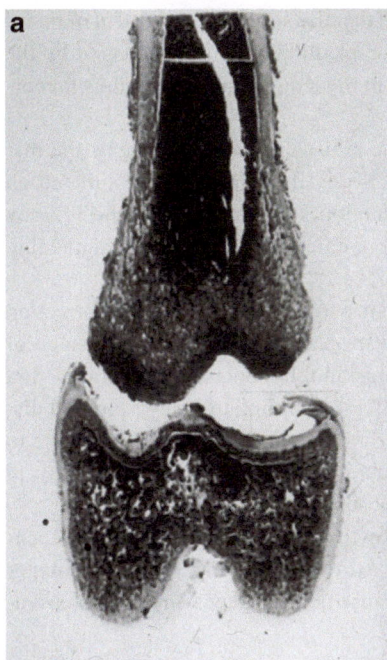

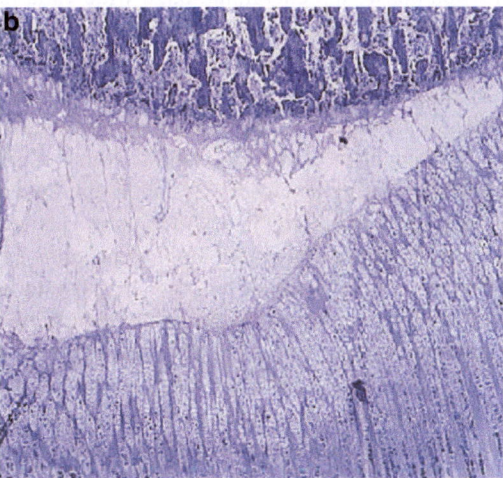

Fig. 4.4 These two histological images of an experimental epiphysiolysis in a lamb show the disruption is produced through the layer of degenerative cells of the growth plate. Most of the growth plate remains together with the epiphysis

period, indicating hyperplasia without bone fracture. During the fracture of epiphyseal cartilage, the forces of distraction reached 80–150 kPa[33–35] or 28–58 kg/m^2.[12] Tercedor et al[59] observed that in all physeal distractions there is an initial hyperplasic reaction in all the cell layers of the growth cartilage, followed by atrophy.

Physeal Distraction in Orthopaedic Surgery

Progressive lengthening is currently a common therapeutic method. Its history can be traced back to pioneering work in 1905 by Codivilla,[10] whose technique was successively modified to make it simpler and more convenient for the patient, reducing the length of treatment, and the incidence of complications. The forerunners of the techniques in use today were developed by Anderson,[3] who has often been unjustly overlooked; he made a general practice of percutaneous osteotomy, thereby avoiding open surgery and the corresponding soft tissue damage and possible complications.

After a period in which the poor results of earlier techniques led to the abandonment of lengthening as a therapeutic method, Wagner[62] proposed a new technique which served to re-establish the method. Wagner's technique only enjoyed a short period of popularity, however, as its introduction coincided with the propagation in the West of Ilizarov's[24–25] ideas which, in principle, rendered long stays in hospital unnecessary.

Ilizarov[24,26] developed the concept of corticotomy, thereby solving the problem of maintaining bone continuity. Both the periosteum and the medulla remain undamaged by the osteotomy, which ensures improved vascularisation in the lengthening callus, thus favouring its regeneration.

With Ilizarov's[24] method the consolidation phase is usually twice as long as the distraction phase. In general, although wide variation is possible, duration is estimated on the basis of 1 month per centimetre of increased length. The drawback of the Ilizarov technique is that the apparatus used is bulky and inconvenient where bilateral lengthening is required.

There are three cases in which physeal distraction is particularly effective: in correction of dissymmetries of the lower limbs which are not in excess of 10% once the stage of growth is nearing its close[2,11,33–35]; in progressive congenital hypoplasia during the period of intense growth[12]; and in achondroplastic patients.[14,15] According to Paley[40] physeal distraction produces more rapid ossification, allows earlier weight-loading, and gives rise to fewer complications than do other lengthening techniques but should be used only in children over 12, owing to the risk of premature closure of the epiphysis. According to Bjerkreim,[5] despite the risk of adversely affecting growth cartilage, which requires suspension of lengthening until growth is complete, physeal distraction has many advantages when compared with lengthening by osteotomy because neither osteotomy and osteosynthesis nor bone grafts are needed (Fig. 4.5).

At present, we accept the following indications for physeal distraction of the distal extreme of the femur or the proximal end of the tibia (a) small dissymmetry, (b) congenital short femur, (c) dissymmetry with dysplasia of the hip, (d) dissymmetry with angular correction and (e) metaphyseal bone tumours.

Technical Aspects of Physeal Distraction with a Unilateral External Fixator

The external fixator is of proven effectiveness in the treatment of fractures. As a consequence of direct experience, development and new designs, the indications for the external fixator have broadened far beyond the original basic indications. Nowadays, the external fixator is used by many departments in the treatment of limb fractures, as well as in cases of retarded consolidation, pseudoarthrosis, axial corrections and in limb lengthening.

The ideal degree of rigidity exerted by an external fixator is unknown at present. On the basis of our experience, the stability of the external fixator should, at the outset, be greater than that of the bone. The stability can later be gradually reduced so that the weight of the load can be transmitted directly to the callus, thus stimulating bone formation.

When using an external fixator, a number of technical aspects should be considered to obtain good results. Surgical intervention using the external fixator should be performed as corrective surgery and carefully planned to accomodate the technical specifications of the apparatus being used.

The surgical technique is straightforward. The mobility of the pinclamps and the fact that the length of the bar can be adjusted facilitate use of the fixator. Once the size of fixator to be used has been chosen, the apparatus is placed alongside the bone which is to be lengthened and adjusted according to the specific measurements of the particular bone.

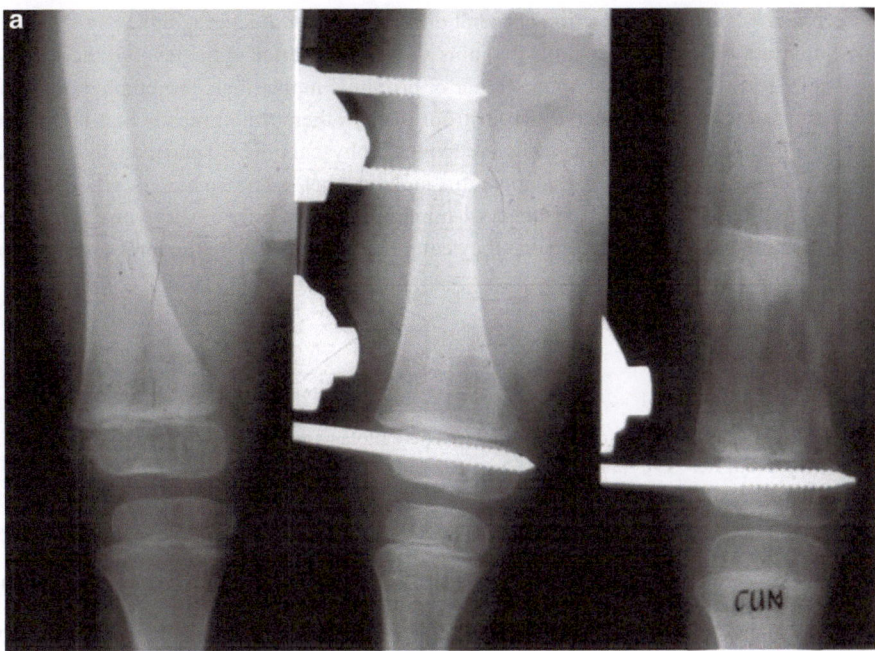

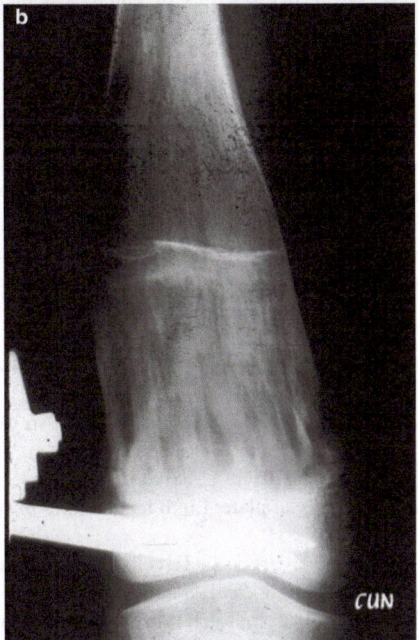

Fig. 4.5 Physeal distraction has been widely used in orthopaedics as a bone lengthening procedure

Technically, physeal distraction does not differ greatly from lengthening procedure: the only important difference is that the two pins should be inserted at the level of the epiphysis, this frequently being distal in the femur or proximal in the tibia. The epiphyseal space requires that the pins be inserted one in front of the other, which means that these pins should be inserted perpendicularly relative to the diaphyseal pins. To carry out this particular procedure, all models of fixator apparatus include what is known as a T-piece.

Pins should be 5 or 6 mm in diameter (4-mm pins are used only in very young children) and care should be taken to ensure that they enter neither too close to the joint cartilage nor too close to the growing cartilage.

References

1. Aldegheri R, Renzi Brivio L, Agostini S. The callotasis method of limb lengthening. *Clin Orthop Relat Res*. 1989;241:137–145.
2. Aldegheri R, Trivella G, Lavini F. Epiphyseal distraction. Chondrodiastasis. *Clin Orthop Relat Res*. 1989;241:117–127.
3. Anderson WV. Leg lengthening. *J Bone Joint Surg*. 1952;34:150–153.
4. Bacci G, Picci P, Pignatti G, et al. Neoadjuvant chemotherapy for nonmetastatic osteosarcoma of the extremities. *Clin Orthop Relat Res*. 1991;270:87–98.
5. Bjerkreim L. Limb lengthening by physeal distraction. *Acta Orthop Scand*. 1989;60:140–142.
6. Bright RW, Elmore SM. Physical properties of epiphyseal plate cartilage. *Surg Forum*. 1968;19:463–465.
7. Brighton CT. The growth plate. *Orthop Clin North Am*. 1984;15:571–595.
8. Bünger C. Hemodynamics of the juvenile knee. *Acta Orthop Scand*. 1987;222:58.
9. Cañadell J, Cara JA, Ganoza C. Physeal distraction and bone lengthening in the conservative treatment of malignant bone tumors in children. In: Cañadell J, Sierrasesúmaga L, Calvo F, Ganoza C, eds. *Treatment of Malignant Bone Tumors in Children and Adolescents*. Pamplona: Servicio de Publicaciones de la, Universidad de Navarra; 1991:293–305.
10. Codivilla A. On the means of lengthening in the lower limbs, the muscles and the tissues which are shortened through deformity. *Am J Orthop Surg*. 1905;2:353–369.
11. Connolly JF, Huurman WW, Lippello L, Pankaj R. Epiphyseal traction to correct acquired growth deformities. *Clin Orthop Relat Res*. 1986;202:258–268.
12. Crawford EJ, Jones CB, Dewar ME, Aichroth PM. The force required to rupture the epiphysis in children undergoing epiphyseal leg lengthening. In: *XVII World Congress of SICOT, Munich*; 16–21 Agosto 1985.
13. Dale GG, Harris WR. Prognosis of epiphyseal separation. An experimental study. *J Bone Joint Surg Br*. 1958;40B:116–122.
14. De Bastiani G, Aldegheri R, Renzi-Brivio L, Trivella G. Chondrodiastasis. Controlled symmetrical distraction of the epiphyseal plate. Limb lengthening in children. *J Bone Joint Surg Br*. 1986;66B:550–556.
15. De Bastiani G, Aldegheri R, Renzi-Brivio L, Trivella G. Limb lengthening by distraction of the epiphyseal plate. *J Bone Joint Surg Br*. 1986;66B:545–549.
16. De Pablos J, Cañadell J. Experimental physeal distraction in immature sheep. *Clin Orthop Relat Res*. 1990;250:73–80.
17. De Pablos J, Villas C, Cañadell J. Bone lengthening by physeal distraction. An experimental study. *Int Orthop*. 1986;10:163–170.
18. Dearden LC. Glucocorticoid effects on the ultrastructure of epiphyseal cartilage. In: Bonucci E, Motta PM, eds. *Ultrastructure of Skeletal Tissue*. Dordecht: Kluwer; 1990.

19. Fishbane BM, Riley LH. Continous transphyseal traction: experimental observations. *Clin Orthop Relat Res*. 1978;136:120–124.

20. Fjeld TO, Steen H. Limb lengthening by low rate epiphyseal distraction. An experimental study in the caprine tibia. *J Orthop Res*. 1988;6:360–368.

21. Gebhardt MC, Flugstad DI, Springfield DS, Mankin HJ. The use of bone allografts for limb salvage in high-grade extremity osteosarcoma. *Clin Orthop Relat Res*. 1991;270:181–196.

22. Harris HA. Bone growth in health an disease. Oxford University Press, Londen, 1933.

23. Hutchinson WJ, Burdeaux BD. The influence of stasis on bone growth. *Surg Gynecol Obstet*. 1954;99:413–420.

24. Ilizarov GA, Soybelman LM. Some clinical and experimental data on the bloodless lengthening of the lower limbs. *Eksp Khir Anesteziol*. 1969;4:27–32.

25. Ilizarov GA. The tension-stress effect on the genesis and growth tissue. Part I. The influence of stability of fixation and soft tissue preservation. *Clin Orthop Relat Res*. 1989;238:249.

26. Ilizarov GA. The tension-stress effect on the genesis and growth tissue. Part II. The influence of the rate and frequency of distraction. *Clin Orthop Relat Res*. 1989;239:263–285.

27. Jani L. Tierexperimentelle Studie über Tibiaverlängerung durch Distrak-tionepiphyseolyse. *Z Orthop*. 1973;111:627–630.

28. Jani L. Die Distraktionepiphyseolyse: Tierexperimentelle Studie zum Problem der Beinverlängerung. *Z Orthop*. 1975;113:189–198.

29. Jee WSS. The skeletal tissues. In: Weiss L, ed., Cell and Tissue Biology. Baltimore: Urban&Schwarzenberg; 1988:213–253.

30. Kuijpers-Jagtman AM, Maltha JC, Bex JHM, Daggers JG. The influence of vascular and periosteal interferences on the histological structure of the growth plates of long bones. *Anat Anz*. 1987;164:245–254.

31. Langenskiöld A. Inhibition and stimulation of growth. *Acta Orthop Scand*. 1957;26:308–316.

32. Letts RM, Meadows L. Epiphysiolysis as a method of limb lengthening. *Clin Orthop Relat Res*. 1978;133:230–237.

33. Monticelli G, Spinelli R. Distraction epiphysiolysis as a method of limb lengthening. III. Clinical applications. *Clin Orthop Relat Res*. 1981;154:274–285.

34. Monticelli G, Spinelli R. Distraction epiphysiolysis as a method of limb lengthening. I. Experimental study. *Clin Orthop Relat Res*. 1981;154:254–261.

35. Monticelli G, Spinelli R. Distraction epiphysiolysis as a method of limb lengthening. II. Morphologic investigations. *Clin Orthop Relat Res*. 1981;154:262–273.

36. Nakamura K, Matsushita T, Okazaki H, Nagano A, Kurokawa T. Attempted limb lengthening by physeal distraction. *Clin Orthop Relat Res*. 1991;267:306–311.

37. Ogihara Y, Ogihara Y, Sudo A, Fujinami S, Sato K. Limb salvage for bone sarcoma of the proximal tibia. *Int Orthop*. 1991;15(4):377–379.

38. Oliete V. Epifisiolisis traumática experimental. Tesis Doctoral. Pamplona: Universidad de Navarra, 1984.

39. Ortiz-Cruz E, Gebhart MC, Hennings LC, Springfield DS, Mankin H. The results of transplantation of intercalary allografts after resection of tumors. A long-term follow-up study. *J Bone Joint Surg Am*. 1997;79(1):97–106.

40. Paley D. Current technique of limb lenghening. *J Pediatr Orthop*. 1988;8:73–92.

41. Peltonen J, Alitalo I, Karaharju EO, Helio H. Distraction of the growth plate: experiments in pigs and sheep. *Acta Orthop Scand*. 1984;55:359–362.

42. Pietravissa G. I distachi epifisari traumatici. *Arch Putti di Chir Org Mov*. 1957;8:153–192.

43. Poole AR, Matsui Y, Hinek A, Lee ER. Cartilage macromolecules and the calcification of cartilage matrix. *Anat Rec*. 1989;224:167–179.

44. Quacci D, DellOrbo C, Pazzaglia UE. Morphological aspects of rat metaphyseal cartilage pericellular matrix. *J Anat*. 1990;171:193–205.

45. Rang M. Childrens fractures. Philadelphia, Toronto: JB Lippincott Co, 1982.
46. Ring PA. Experimental bone lengthening by epiphyseal distraction. *Br J Surg.* 1958;46:169–173.
47. Robertson WW. Newest knowledge of the growth plate. *Clin Orthop Relat Res.* 1990;253: 270–278.
48. Rougraff BT, Rougraff BT, Simon MA, Kneisl JS, Greenberg DB, Mankin HJ. Limb salvage compared with amputation for osteosarcoma of the distal end of the femur. A long-term oncological, functional and quality-of-life study. *J Bone Jt Surg Am.* 1994;75:649–656.
49. Salter RB, Harris WR. Injuries involving the epiphyseal plate. *J Bone Jt Surg Am.* 1963;45:587–622.
50. San Julian M. Recambios protésicos de cadera y rodilla en cirugía tumoral. *Rev Ortop Traumatol.* 2000;44:237–249.
51. Sheldon H, Robinson RA. Studies on rickets. I. The fine structure of uncalcified bone matrix in experimental rickets. *Z Zellforsch Mikrosk Anat.* 1961;53:671–684.
52. Simon MA, Aschliman MA, Thomas N, Mankin HJ. Limb salvage treatment versus amputation for osteosarcoma of the distal end of the femur. *J Bone J Surg Am.* 1986;68:1331–1337.
53. Skak SV, Jensen TT, Poulsen TD, Stürup J. Epidemiology of knee injuries in children. *Acta Orthop Scand.* 1987;58:78–81.
54. Sledge CB, Noble J. Experimental limb lengthening by epiphyseal distraction. *Clin Orthop Relat Res.* 1978;136:111.
55. Sola CK, Silberman FS, Cabrini RL. Stimulation of the longitudinal growth of long bones by periosteal stripping. *J Bone Joint Surg Am.* 1963;45A:1679–1684.
56. Springgins AJ, Bader DL, Cunningham JL, Kenwright J. Distraction physiolysis in the rabbit. *Acta Orthop Scand.* 1989;60(2):154–158.
57. Steen H, Fjeld TO, Ronningen H, Langeland N, Gjerdet N, Bjerkreim I. Limb lengthening by epiphyseal distraction. An experimental study in the caprine femur. *J Orthop Res.* 1987;5:592–599.
58. Taillard W, Morscher E. Die Beinlängeunterschiede. Basel, New York: Karger, 1965.
59. Tercedor J, Crespo V, Acosta F, Campos A, Fernandez E. Alargamiento tibial por distracción epifisaria proximal. Estudio experimental en conejos. *Rev Ortop Traumatol.* 1988;32IB:412–416.
60. Trueta J. The influence of the blood supply in controlling bone growth. *Bull Hosp Jt Dis.* 1953;14:147–157.
61. Trueta J, Amato VP. The vascular contribution to osteogenesis. III. Changes in the growth cartilage caused by experimentally induced ischaemia. *J Bone Joint Surg Br.* 1960;42:571–587.
62. Wagner M. Opertive Beinverlängerung. *Chirurg.* 1971;42:260–266.
63. Weber BG, Brunner C, Freuler F. Treatment of fractures in children and adolescents. Berlin, Heidelberg, New York: Springer, 1980.
64. Zavijalov PV, Plaskin JT. Elongation of crural bones in children using a method of distraction epiphysiolysis. *Vestn Khir Im I I Grek.* 1967;103:67.

A Histological Study of the Barrier Effect of the Physis Against Metaphyseal Osteosarcoma

5

Miguel Angel Idoate, Enrique de Alava, Julio de Pablos,
Maria Dolores Lozano, Jesús Vazquez, and José Cañadell

Abstract In half the children affected by metaphyseal malignant bone tumours, the physis and epiphysis are not compromised by the tumour. Invasion of the epiphysis by the tumour seems to be a matter of time.

Introduction

Osteosarcoma is a primary malignant bone tumour usually located in the metaphysis. It tends to infiltrate adjacent bone as well as soft tissue.

Traditionally, the physis has been regarded as a barrier capable of preventing tumour extension.[1,5] This idea has been strengthened by experimental studies carried out in vitro which attribute this characteristic of the physis to certain inhibitory protein substances of angiogenesis.[2,10,11] However, the physeal invasion observed in skeletally immature patients with osteogenic sarcoma[4,7,9,13,14] raises doubts about the barrier function.

It is important to establish the frequency with which osteosarcoma invades the physis. Knowledge of this frequency helps not only in assessing tumour extension but also in planning surgical resection.

In this study, which we carried out many years ago, 24 cases of osteosarcoma in skeletally immature patients were reviewed with the objective of clarifying how effective the physis is as a barrier to tumour spread. An additional objective was to define types of physeal invasion and correlate these with radiological findings.

Materials and Methods

The study covers 24 surgically resected specimens diagnosed by biopsies from 1979 to 1986, at the beginning of the "chemotherapy era." In order to ascertain tumour extension reliably at the time of diagnosis, all cases had been studied by conventional radiology, computerised axial tomography (CT), and digital angiography.

Miguel Angel Idoate (✉)
Department of Pathology, University Clinic of Navarra, Avda. Pio XII 38, Pamplona,
Navarrav 31080, Spain
e-mail: maidoate@unav.es

J. Cañadell and M. San-Julian (eds.), *Pediatric Bone Sarcomas: Epiphysiolysis Before Excision*,
DOI: 10.1007/978-1-84882-130-9_5, © Springer-Verlag London Limited 2011

After histological diagnosis and prior to surgical resection, all patients but one received adjuvant chemotherapy, with the selective agent cisplatin administered through the arteries supplying the tumour and Adriamycin administered intravenously. According to the type of surgical treatment, the cases were divided into two groups:

Group I: 19 patients in whom conservative surgery was applied without physeal preservation. In 16 cases, the primary tumour was located in the distal *femur*, in two cases in the proximal *humerus* and in one case in the proximal *femur*. Twelve patients were females and 7 males. Mean age was 13 years, the range being between 9 and 17 years

Group II: Five patients whose tumours were resected by conservative surgery with physeal and epiphyseal preservation after physeal distraction. In these five cases, the epiphysis had not been affected by the tumour and this was established beyond doubt with the above-mentioned imaging methods and confirmed by epiphyseal biopsies. This group was composed of three females and two males, with a mean age of 12 years (ranging from 8 to 14 years). In all cases, the tumours were located in the distal *femur*.

The specimens obtained by resection were studied macroscopically and microscopically. In all cases, the stains applied were the H&E stain and Masson's trichrome stain. Multiple sections were taken from the metaphyseal area and, when included in the resection, from physeal and epiphyseal areas.

___

Results

The osteosarcomas were of the following histological types: osteoblastic (19), chondroblastic (4), and fibroblastic (1).

The tumour tissue, as a result of the pre-operative chemotherapeutic treatment, always presented a highly altered histological picture at the time of resection. In some cases, there was only a dense mass of post-necrotic connective scar tissue within which histologically normal bone *trabeculae* could sometimes be seen.

Physeal invasion was observed in the resection specimens from 12 of the 19 patients of Group I (61.1%). Of these, epiphyseal invasion was observed in 11. None of the metaphyseal resection margins in the specimens from the five cases in Group II (treated by physeal distraction) was affected by tumour. Considering all the cases together (Group I and Group II), epiphyseal invasion was observed in 50% of patients.

With regard to age, note that the average age at the time of tumour resection was 14.5 years for patients with epiphyseal involvement but 12.5 for patients without.

We observed three morphological pictures of tumour and physis. In 12 cases, between the tumour and the physis, there was a metaphyseal band of variable width (2–10 mm) within which there was no detectable neoplastic disease. This disease-free metaphyseal zone had increased vascularization, consisting of ectatic capillaries, and numerous osteoclastic cells flanking bone *trabeculae*, whose surfaces appeared undulate (Fig. 5.1).

In one case, the tumour made contact with the physis, on the metaphyseal side. In the zone of contact, the physis appeared uniformly thinned, the hypertrophic and calcification zones having practically disappeared.

The third morphological picture was seen in the remaining 11 cases, where epiphyseal tumour invasion was observed. Morphologically there were two patterns of physeal

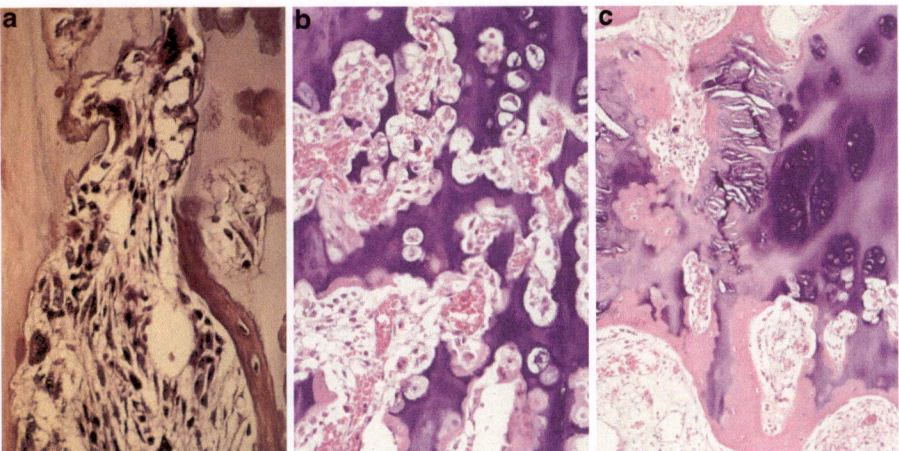

Fig. 5.1 Osteoclastic activation accompanying fibrovascular proliferation in the femoral physis of a 10-year-old osteosarcoma patient. The front edge of tumour front extends upwards to 4 mm from the physis, which remains un-invaded (H&E ×200)

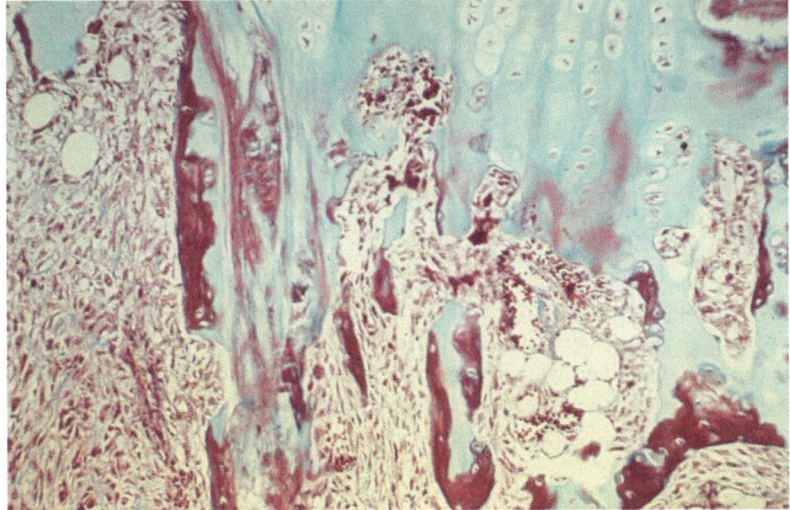

Fig. 5.2 Physeal invasion by an osteosarcoma in a 12-year-old male. Tumour cells invade infiltrate as finger-like growths permeating the calcification and hypertrophic zones of the physeal cartilage. (Masson's trichrome ×40)

invasion. In the first pattern, epiphyseal areas were in close contact with the tumour but not completely invaded by it. Tumour cells could be seen permeating the spaces between cartilaginous matrix columns; capillaries were dilated (Fig. 5.2). In the second pattern, in addition to the changes indicated above, there was perforation and thinning of the growth cartilage. The perforation was multi-focal, leaving dispersed islands of highly disorganized cartilage within the tumour tissue (Fig. 5.3).

Fig. 5.3 Remains of physeal cartilage in the femur of an 8-year-old girl with metaphyseal osteoblastic osteosarcoma. The patient had received chemotherapy before resection of the tumour. Islands of physeal cartilage can be seen surrounded by reparative tissue which occupies the whole thickness of the physis after having substituted necrotic tumour (H&E ×100)

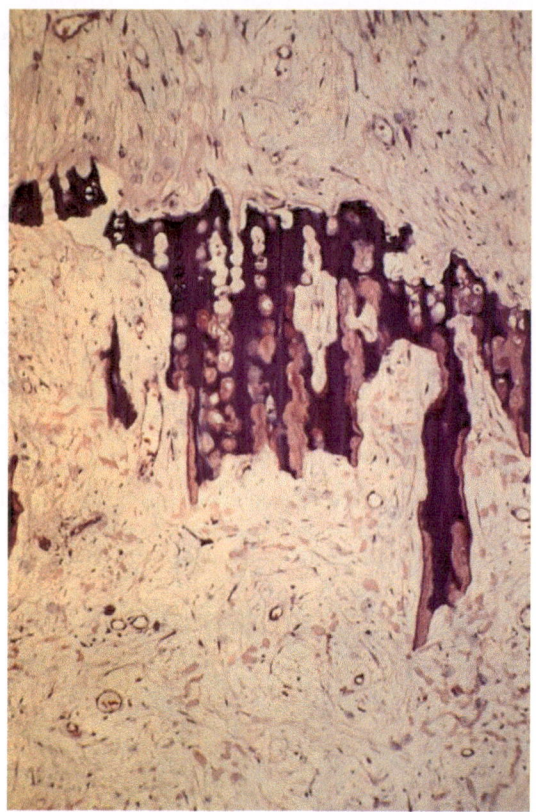

In general, the extensions of tumour into the epiphysis appeared to have expanded evenly (Fig. 5.4). Some sections revealed paradoxical areas in which neoplastic tissue appeared on both sides of growth cartilage; the apparent lack of connection can be explained by supposing that the plane of section did not cross the area of physeal involvement by the tumour (Fig. 5.5).

Discussion

The frequency of epiphyseal invasion in our series, 12 of 24 (50%), is lower than that of previous reports: Enneking and Kagan[7] found 17 of 24 cases (70.8%) to have transphyseal tumour invasion towards the epiphysis; Norton et al.[13] found epiphyseal invasion in 12 of 15 cases (80%); Simon and Bos,[14] 23 of 26 (88.5%); and Ghandur-Mnaymneh et al,[9] 12 of 14 (85.7%).

In a recent case (Fig. 5.6), we had the opportunity to analyze two consecutive MR images for a patient who did not receive any treatment for his tumour for over a month. The two images also suggest that invasion of the physis is a matter of time.

Fig. 5.4 Physeal tumour invasion, in the form of finger-like projections, which respects the adjacent physis in a 9-year-old female with osteoblastic osteosarcoma. The periphery of the osteosarcoma was not necrotic despite pre-operative chemotherapy. This multi-focal type of growth is more difficult to detect radiologically (H&E ×100)

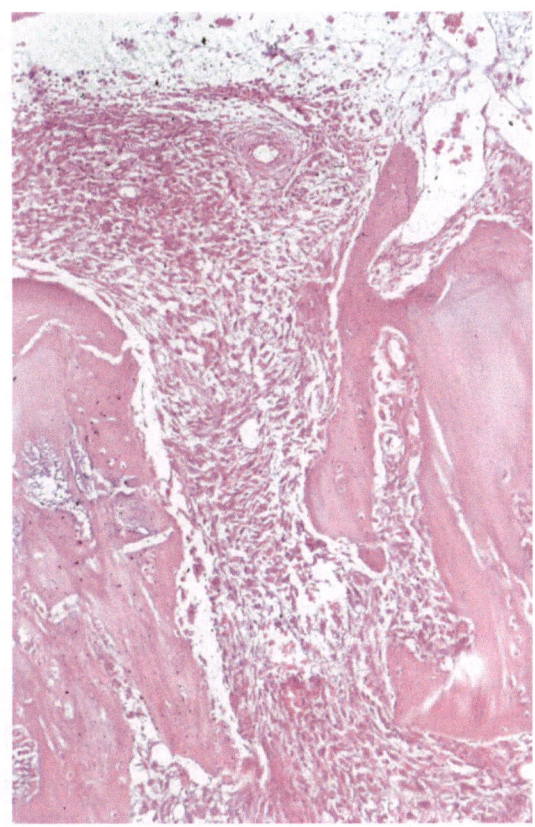

The percentage of patients with epiphyseal invasion, although less than those of previous reports, is still very significantly greater than zero, and this must surely raise doubts about the traditional notion of the "physeal barrier." If the physis does not represent an impenetrable barrier, then it is possible that physeal invasion by any metaphyseal osteosarcoma is a matter of time. In this case, earlier diagnosis might be responsible for the lower percentage of physeal-epiphyseal invasion in our series with respect to others.

There is no clear relationship between the histological type of an osteosarcoma and its capacity for epiphyseal invasion.

Two main theories have been proposed to explain how osteosarcoma, in its spread, is able to cross the physis.[14] According to the first, epiphyseal invasion takes place through the pre-existing transphyseal vascular channels, which communicate the metaphysis with the epiphysis.[7,15] However, Trueta and Morgan[16] and Brighton[3] observed that, from approximately 1.5–2 years of life until the age of skeletal maturity, the human epiphyseal and metaphyseal circulations are not connected in any way through the physis, which is hypertrophic. Most proliferating cartilage is practically avascular.

The second theory is based on the possibility that the tumour induces an intense vascular response at its periphery, which favours its spread.[8] Our findings are concordant with such a mechanism. Vascular proliferation of the peritumoural stroma would favour

Fig. 5.5 A paradoxical pattern of metaphyseal-epiphyseal infiltration in which there is apparent preservation of the physis, at least on the plane of this section. From a 15-year-old male with osteosarcoma. (H&E ×100)

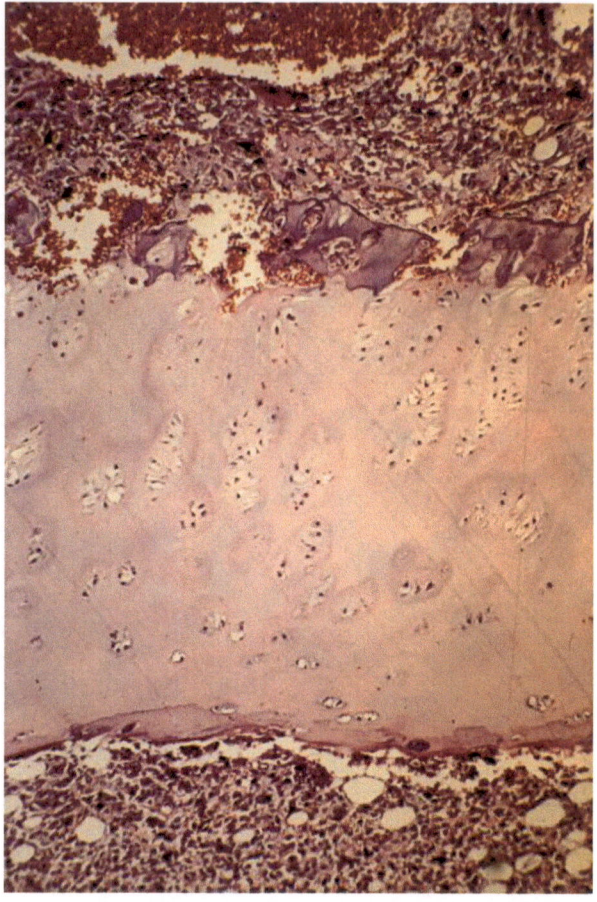

tumour infiltration of the cellular columns of epiphyseal cartilage observed in our histological studies. This infiltration would also be enhanced by the osteoclastic reaction, which was seen in the free zone between the tumour and the physis as a phenomenon that precedes the tumour.

Apart from the transphyseal route of epiphyseal invasion, another explanation of how the tumour gets into the epiphysis is to suppose that it can establish epiphyseal metastatic foci without alterations in the growth cartilage. This type of metastasis, so-called *skip metastasis*, has been observed to occur between various zones of a single bone[6] and even between adjacent bones of mature individuals without affecting the articular cartilage.[12] However, there was no evidence of such metastasis in our histological study.

Age is a factor which one might expect to influence trans-physeal spread of osteosarcoma. Physeal involution commences shortly before skeletal maturity and, as a result of this, at certain points, metaphyso-epiphyseal vascular communication is re-established.

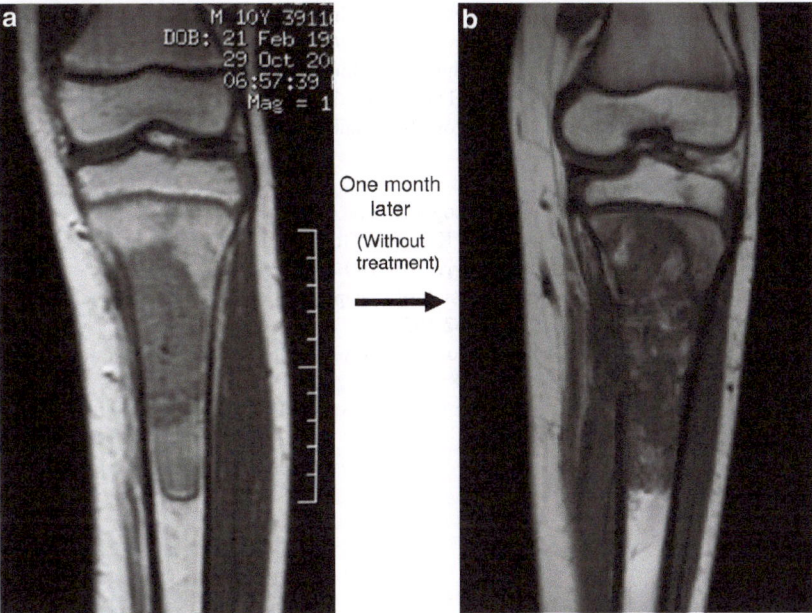

Fig. 5.6 The initial MRI scan for this patient with a bone sarcoma was made at a hospital other than our own. Over a month later, he came to our centre, and we took another MRI scan in order to be sure the epiphysis could still be saved. These two consecutive scans strongly suggest that involvement of the physis is a matter of time.

These changes would increase the possibility of an osteosarcoma invading the epiphysis. In our series, however, although a difference was observed between the age of patients with physeal and/or epiphyseal invasion (14.5 years) with respect to the group without physeal invasion (12.5 years), this difference was not statistically significant.

References

1. Aegerter E, Kirkpatrick J. Orthopaedic diseases. *Physiology, Pathology*. Filadelfia: WB Saunders; 1975:519.
2. Brem H, Folkman J. Inhibition of tumor angiogenesis mediated by cartilage. *J Exp Med*. 1975;141:427.
3. Brighton CT. The growth plate. *Orthop Clin Nort Am*. 1984;15:571.
4. Castiella T. El disco fisario frente al osteosarcoma de localización metafisaria. *Rev Ortop Traum*. 1982;26:301.
5. Dahlin DC. Bone tumors: General aspects and data on 6221 cases. Springfield: Charles C. Thomas; 1978:234.
6. Ennekingg WF, Kagan A. Skip metastasis in osteosarcoma. *Cancer*. 1975;36:2192.
7. Ennekingg WF, Kagan A. Transepiphyseal extension of osteosarcoma: incidence, mechanism and implications. *Cancer*. 1978;41:1526.
8. Folkman J. Tumor angiogenesis: therapeucit implications. *N Engl J Med*. 1971;285:1182.

9. Ghandur-Mnaymneh L, Mnaymneh WA, Puls S. The incidence and mechanism of transphyseal spread of osteosarcoma of long bones. *Clin Orthop*. 1983;177:210.

10. Kuettner KE, Pauli BU, Soble L. Morphological studies on the resistance of cartilage to invasion by osteosarcoma cell "in vitro" and "in vivo." *Cancer Res*. 1978;38:277.

11. Langer R. Isolation of cartilage factor that inhibits tumor neovascularization. *Science*. 1976;193:70.

12. Missenarg GM. Confrontation anatomoclinique pré et postopératoire: á propos de 30 resections conservatrices pour sarcomes osteogènes. *Rev Chir Orthop*. 1986:72:477.

13. Norton KI, Hermann G, Abdelwahab IF, Klein MJ, Granowetter LF, Rabinowitz JG. Epiphyseal involvement in osteosarcoma. *Radiology*. 1991;180:813–816.

14. Simon MA, Bos GD. Epiphyseal extension of metaphyseal osteosarcoma in skeletally immature individuals. *J Bone Jt Surg*. 1980;62:195.

15. Spira E, Farin I. The vascular supply to the epiphyseal plate under normal and pathological conditions. *Acta Orthop Scand*. 1967;38:1.

16. Trueta J, Morgan JD. The vascular contribution to osteogenesis. I. Studies by the injection method. *J Bone Jt Surg*. 1960;42-B:97.

Growth Plate Involvement in Malignant Bone Tumours: Relationship Between Imaging Methods and Histological Findings

6

Jesús Dámaso Aquerreta, Mikel San-Julián, Alberto Benito, and José Cañadell

Abstract MRI is a very reliable imaging method for detecting physeal and epiphyseal involvement in metaphyseal malignant bone tumours. In our experience, we have had no false negatives.

Introduction

In the late 1970s and early 1980s, several advances enabled surgeons to broaden the indications for limb salvage: better and more accurate diagnostic imaging techniques became available,[1–13] techniques of bone reconstruction were improved, there was progress in methods for resection of pulmonary metastases, and above all, pre- and post-operative chemotherapy protocols became established. Limb preserving procedures require knowledge of the exact extension of the tumour, and so, in this chapter, we will consider the role of imaging methods and how accurately and specifically they determine the intraoseous extent of tumours. To this end, we carried out a study comparing several imaging methods that are employed in the evaluation of physeal involvement in primary malignant bone tumours.

Patients and Methods

We analyzed metaphyseal malignant bone tumours in under 16-year-olds treated in our department between 1982 and 1995. Of the 65 tumours studied, 47 were osteosarcomas and 18 Ewing's sarcomas. The mean age of the patients was 11 (3–16) years.

Standard radiographs were available for all patients. Computed tomography (CT) scans were available for 51 patients, digital angiography (Fig. 6.1) images for 48, and magnetic resonance imaging (MRI) T1- and T2-weighted sequences for 31. All methods were evaluated by the same radiologist.

Jesus Dámaso Aquerreta (✉)
Department of Radiology, University Clinic of Navarra, Avda Pio XII, 36, Pamplona, Navarra, 31008, Spain
e-mail: Jdaquerret@unav.es

J. Cañadell and M. San-Julian (eds.), *Pediatric Bone Sarcomas: Epiphysiolysis Before Excision,*   79
DOI: 10.1007/978-1-84882-130-9_6, © Springer-Verlag London Limited 2011

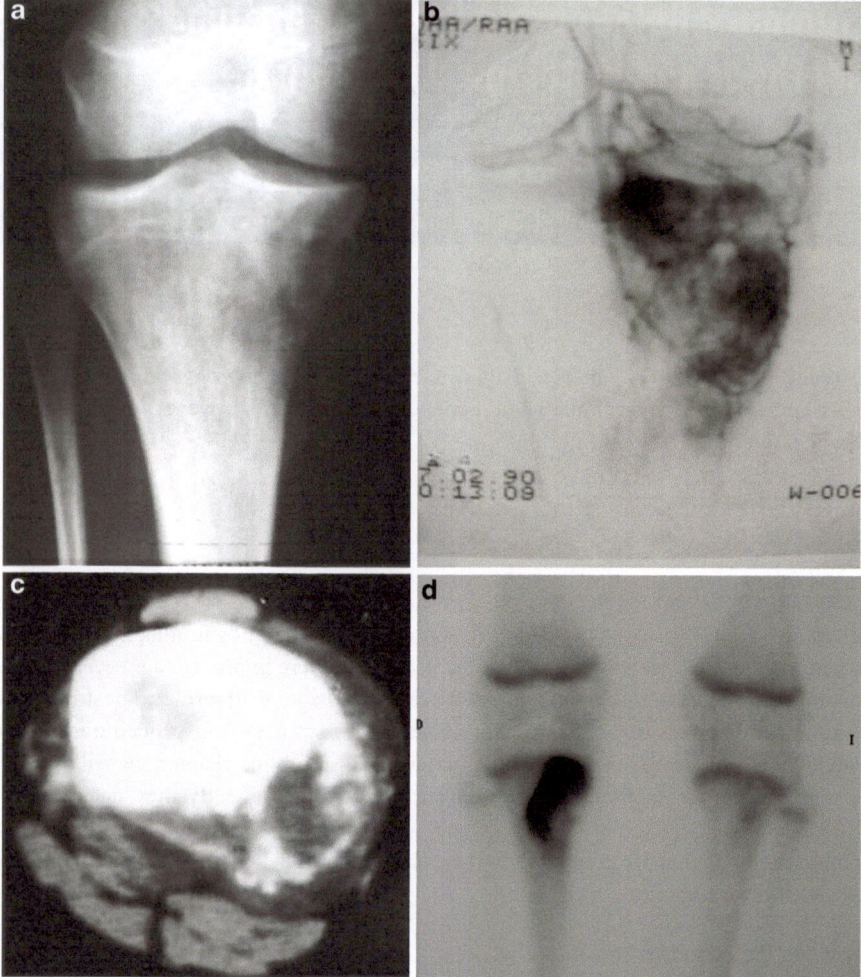

Fig. 6.1 X-ray (**a**), angiography (**b**), and CT (**c**) images used for assessing tumour involvement of the epiphysis. (**d**) A bone scan of a different case showing an epiphysis free of tumour

Careful histological examination of all the resected pieces was performed, especially of the metaphyseal margin in cases in which the epiphysis was preserved.

The proximity of the tumour to the growth plate was evaluated with as many of the different methods as possible. A tumour was considered to be at *distance zero* if it was in contact or had crossed the growth plate. On the basis of the histological findings, we studied the following statistical parameters of the four imaging methods: sensitivity, specificity, accuracy, and positive and negative predictive values.

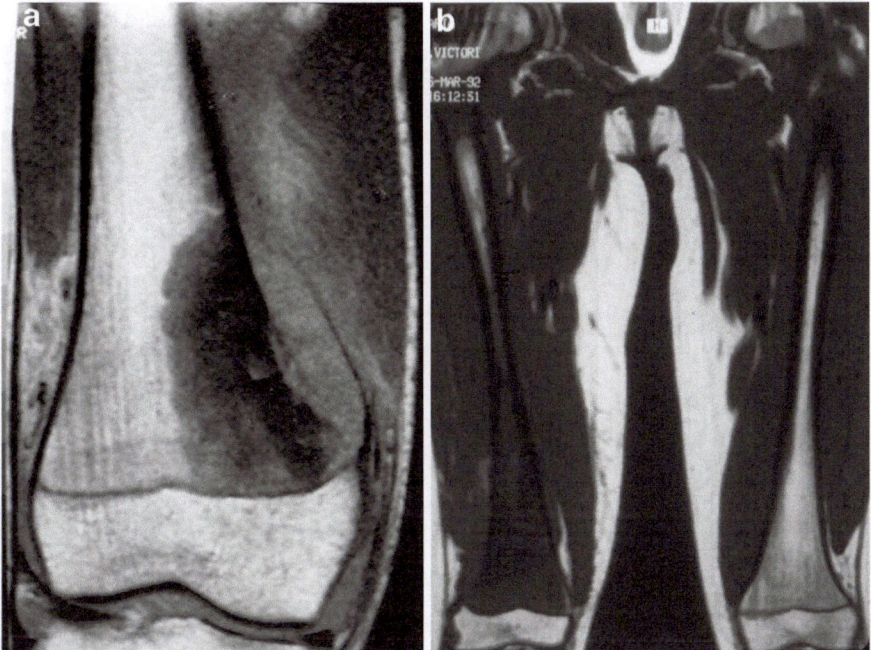

Fig. 6.2 MRI was the best imaging method for assessing tumoural involvement of the growth plate

Results

The physis was affected in 53% of cases (Figs. 6.2 and 6.3). Table 6.1 presents the relationship between histological findings and the evaluation of growth plate involvement based on the different imaging methods.

The sensitivity with CT and MRI was 100%, with X-ray and angiography, over 90%. The specificity with MRI was 78.5%.

Predictive value and accuracy data is given in Table 6.2. The positive predictive value (the probability of actual involvement of the growth plate given that with the imaging method it was *seen* to be involved) was more than 80% for all the methods studied. The negative predictive value (the probability that the imaging method correctly indicated that the growth plate was not involved) was 100% in CT and MRI. The greatest accuracy (the average of the positive and negative predictive values) was obtained with MRI (90.3%).

With MRI, we found that it was possible to distinguish three types of lesion:

- The tumour was not in contact with the growth plate. In some cases, the radiologist could discern oedema between the tumoural lesion and the growth plate, and this was an important feature in determining the surgical approach.

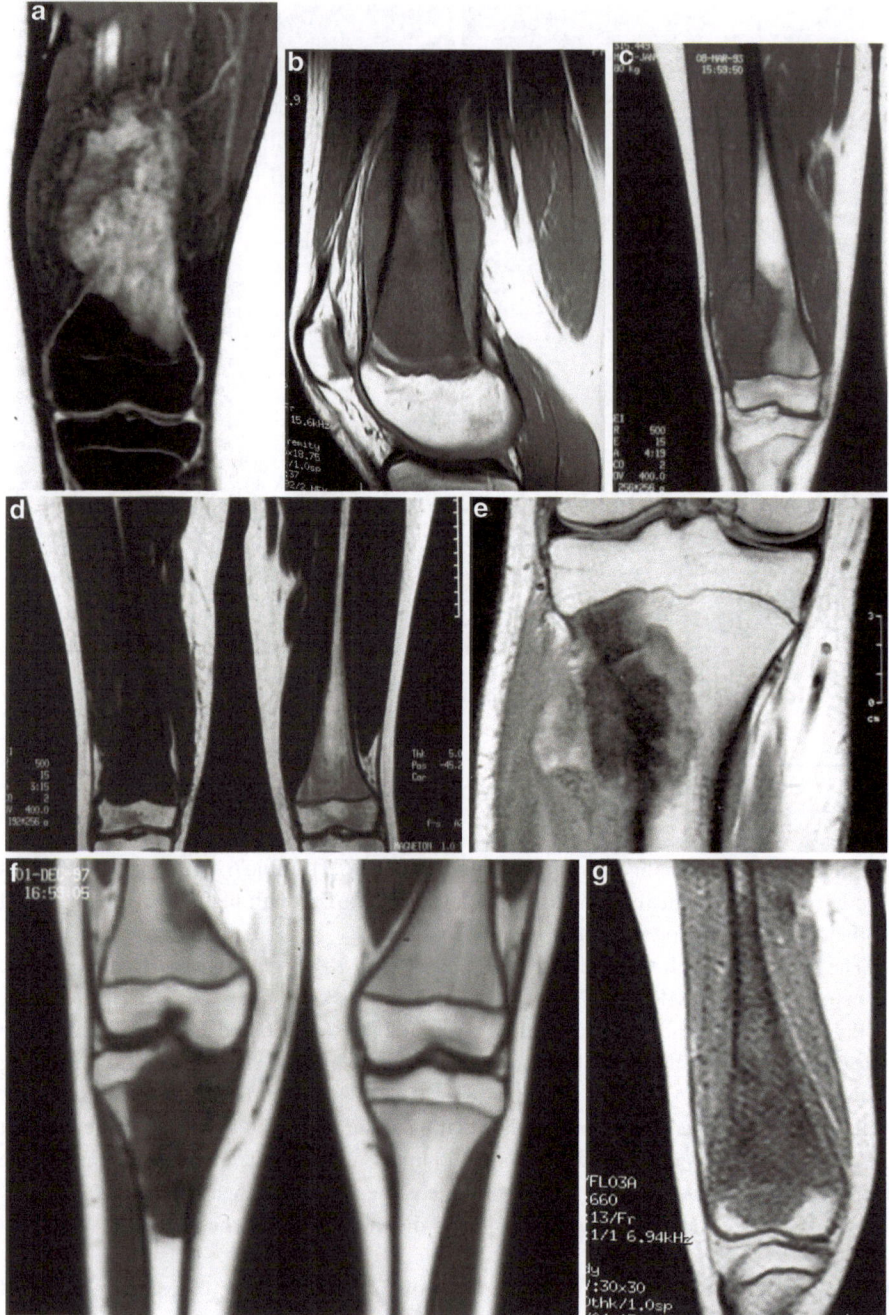

Fig. 6.3 In 50% of the cases (**a–d**), the physis was not crossed by the tumour. In the other cases, the tumour introduced itself into the epiphysis (**f**, **g**)

Table 6.1 Relationship between imaging and histological findings

N° of cases studied with every imaging method	False (−)	False (+)	Total
X-ray (65)	1	6	7 (10.7%)
CT (43)	0	6	6 (13.9%)
Angiography (30)	1	3	4 (13.3%)
MRI (31)	0	3	3 (9.6%)

Table 6.2 Accuracy of the imaging methods

Imaging Method	PPV	NPV	Accuracy
X-ray	82.7	94.7	87.5
CT	81.5	100	86.5
Angiography	85.1	80	84
MRI	87.1	100	90.3

- The tumour was in contact with part or all of the growth plate. In some of these cases, it was possible to resect the tumour while preserving the epiphysis (*see* Chap. 7).
- The tumour transgressed the physis.

Discussion

Despite its general low specificity, over a century of experience with X-ray imaging make it the primary and indispensable methodology for visualization of bone pathologies.

CT can be regarded as a complementary technique to X-ray because it provides better imaging of complex zones such as pelvic bones. A disadvantage of CT is that it does not offer multi-planar images, thus making examination of the growth plate difficult because the physis is not a plane surface.

A technique not included in our study is scintigraphy, which, due to its very high sensitivity, is more generally used in cancer patients to determine whether or not there is multiple bone involvement. For the purpose of evaluating involvement of the growth plate, the low specificity of scintigraphy means it is not particularly useful: in most cases, both the lesion and the growth plate show increased up-take of the radiopharmaceutical (Fig. 6.1d).

Angiography shows the vascular supply to tumours and facilitates staging a tumour. Angiography is also helpful for evaluating the likely effectiveness of intra-arterial chemotherapy, which is useful in the treatment of bone tumours, above all in osteosarcoma. Pre-operative chemotherapy, which initially confirmed the action in vivo of drugs on

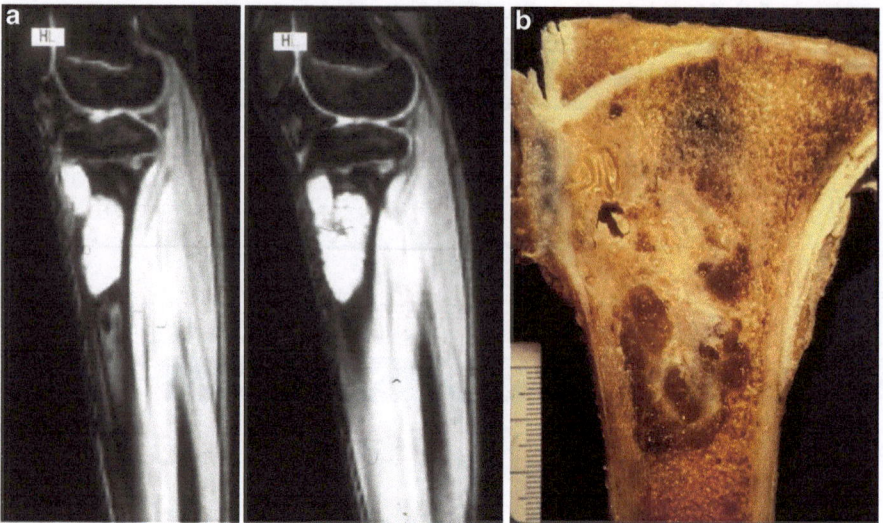

Fig. 6.4 An example of a metaphyseal Ewing's sarcoma that has not crossed the growth plate

tumour tissue, can improve limb preservation. Angiography may also facilitate evaluation of whether or not a tumour has involved the epiphysis, since neovascularization can be observed in this area. With digital subtraction angiography, however, it is more difficult to distinguish bone structures, and thus this method is less useful for the purposes of evaluating growth plate involvement.

In our study, there were more false positive results than false negative ones; with CT and MRI, there were no false negatives. We conclude that, for our purposes, CT and MRI are safe and reliable diagnostic techniques [1–13] (Figs. 6.4 and 6.5).

Although diagnosis should never be based solely on MRI, it is the best available technique for staging a bone tumour because of its high sensitivity and the possibility of multiplanar imaging. MRI provides a clear delineation of tumour extension and shows the association between the tumour and the growth plate. We prefer the T1-weighted image in coronal sections because it enables the use of thin slides with which high contrast between fat and tumour signal intensity can be achieved. The accuracy of this technique in determining physeal involvement was better than that of the others (Figs. 6.1–6.3). Recent data indicate that positron emission tomography could also play an important role in assessing tumoural involvement of the growth plate (Fig. 6.6).

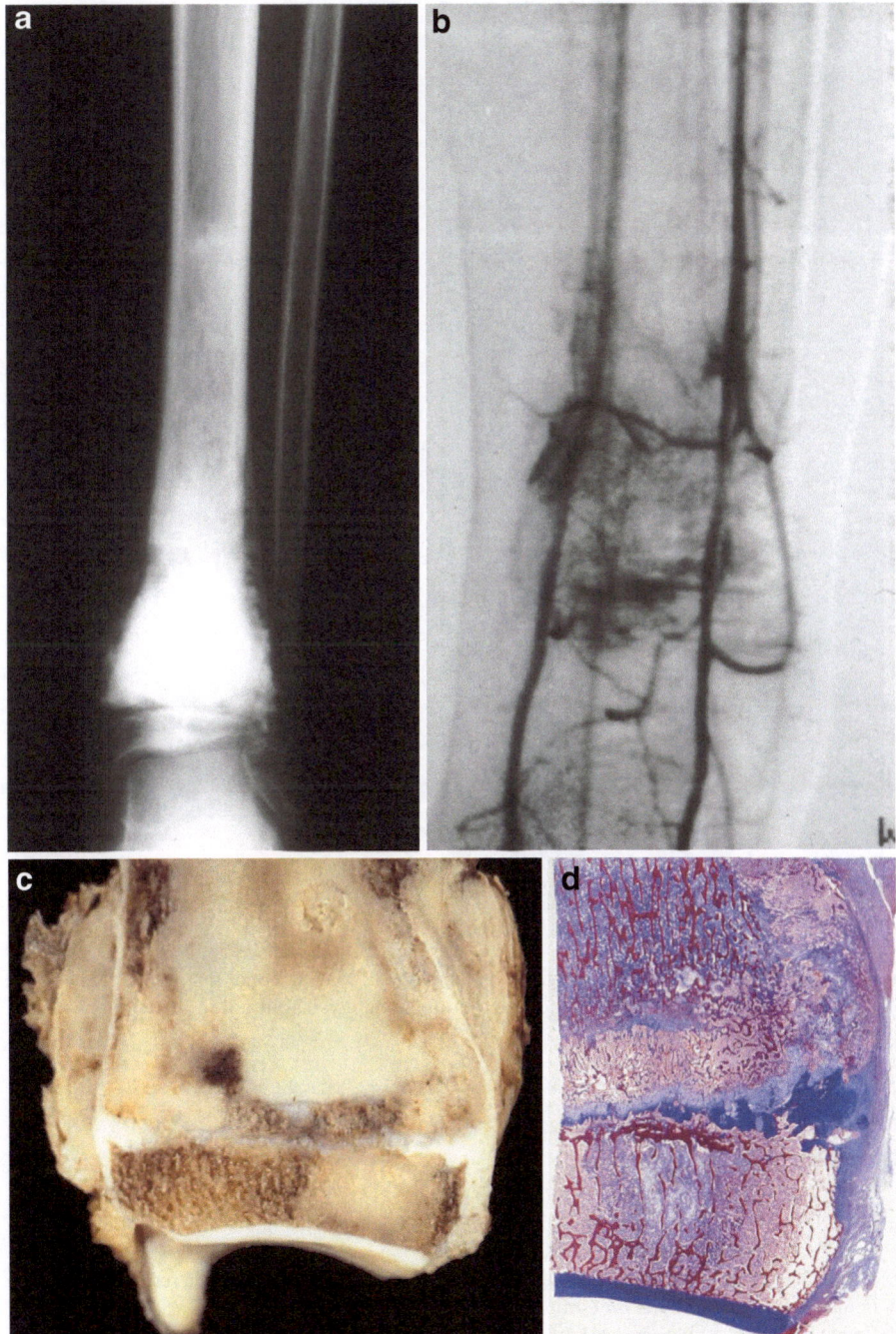

Fig. 6.5 An example of metaphyseal osteosarcoma extending across the growth plate

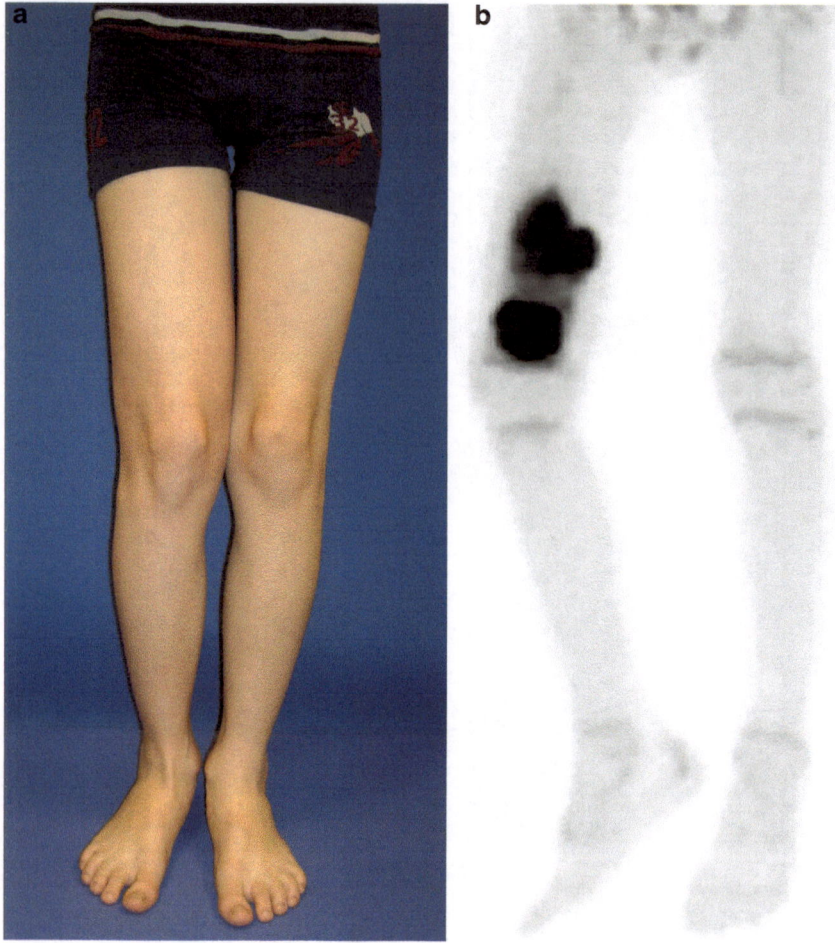

Fig. 6.6 Clinical aspect and PET image of a metaphyseal bone sarcoma that is not crossing the physis. The metabolism of FDG is increased in the metaphysis, but not in the epiphysis. Note the up-take in every growth plate

References

1. Estes DN, Magill HL, Thompson EL, Hayes FA. Primary Ewing's sarcoma: follow up with Ga-67 scintigraphy. *Radiology*. 1990;177:449.
2. Exner GU, Von Hochstetter AR, Augustiny N, Von Schulthess G. Magnetic resonance imaging in malignant bone tumors. *Int Orthop*. 1990;14:49.
3. Frank JA, Ling A, Patronas NJ, et al. Detection of malignant bone tumors: MR imaging vs scintigraphy. *AJR*, 1990;155:1043.
4. Golfieri R, Baddeley H, Pringle JS, Souhami R. The role of the STIR sequence in magnetic resonance imaging examination of bone tumors. *Br J Radiol*. 1990;63:251.

5. Hudson TM, Hamlin DS, Enneking WF, Peterson H. Magnetic resonance imaging of bone and soft tissue tumors. *Skeletal Radiol.* 1985;13:134.
6. Kattapuram SV. Imaging of musculoskeletal tumors. *Curr Opin Orthopaed.* 1991;2:781.
7. Knop J, Delling G, Heise U, Winkler K. Scintigraphic of tumor regression during preoperative chemotherapy of osteosarcoma: correlation of Tc-99m-methylene diphosphonate parametric imaging with surgical histopathology. *Skeletal Radiol.* 1990;19:165.
8. Lemmi MA, Fletcher RB, Marina NM, et al. Use of L MR imaging to assess results of chemotherapy for Ewing sarcoma. *AJR.* 1990;155:343.
9. O'Flanagan SJ, Stack JP, Mccee HM, Dervan P, Hurson B. Imaging of intramedullary tumor spread in osteosarcoma: a comparison of techniques. *J Bone Joint Surg (Am).* 1991;73-A:998-1001.
10. San Julian M, Aquerreta JD, Benito A, Cañadell J. Indications for epiphyseal preservation in metaphyseal malignant bone tumors of children. Relationship between image methods and anatomopathological findings *Am J Pediatr Orthopaedics* 1999;19:543-548.
11. Sundaram M, McLeod RA. MR imaging of tumor and tumor-like lesions of bone and soft tissue. *AJR.* 1990;155:817.
12. Vander Griend RA, Eenneking WF. Radiologic imaging techniques in the diagnosis and treatment of osteogenic sarcoma. *Semin Orthop.* 1988;3:59.
13. Zimmer WD, Berquist TH, McLeod RA, et al. Bone tumors: magnetic resonance imaging versus computer tomography. *Radiology.* 1985;155:709.

Imaging-Based Indications for Resection with Epiphyseal Preservation

7

Mikel San-Julian and José Cañadell

Abstract The findings of imaging methods can be used to select cases in which we can try to preserve the epiphysis during tumour resection.

Introduction

On the basis of the findings of the various imaging methods considered in Chap. 3, we can identify cases in which the tumour does not involve the epiphysis and in these cases, adopt an approach to tumour resection which attempts to preserve the epiphysis. Such an approach involves a carefully coordinated chemotherapy programme before resection, with the aim of minimising the risk of local recurrence.

We carried out a study comparing several imaging methods that are employed in the evaluation of physeal involvement in primary malignant bone tumours. By correlating our findings with the histological features of each case, we were able to establish indications for our technique of epiphyseal preservation through physeal distraction (epiphysiolysis) before excision of metaphyseal bone tumours in children.[1]

In our imaging study (Chap. 6), there were more false positive than false negative results; in the CT and MRI studies, there were no false negatives which confirms that MRI and CT scan are safe and reliable diagnostic techniques that allow us to predict the location and extent of a tumour and, where oncologically appropriate, reduce the amount of bone resected.[3–14] The problem of false positives with CT and MRI (Fig. 7.1), however, could lead us to a sub-optimal treatment of certain tumours.

Several years ago, in our department, we carried out a retrospective histological study of a series of malignant bone tumours in children[2] (*see* Chap. 5). The proportion of cases in which the tumour infringed the physis, about 50%, was similar to that found with our subsequent study of imaging methods (*see* Chap. 6). In the histological study, we found that morphological lesions at the physis could be categorized into three types:

Mikel San-Julian (✉)
Department of Orthopedic Surgery, University Clinic of Navarra, Avda. Pio XII, s/n,
Pamplona, Navarra, 31008, Spain

J. Cañadell and M. San-Julian (eds.), *Pediatric Bone Sarcomas: Epiphysiolysis Before Excision*,
DOI: 10.1007/978-1-84882-130-9_7, © Springer-Verlag London Limited 2011

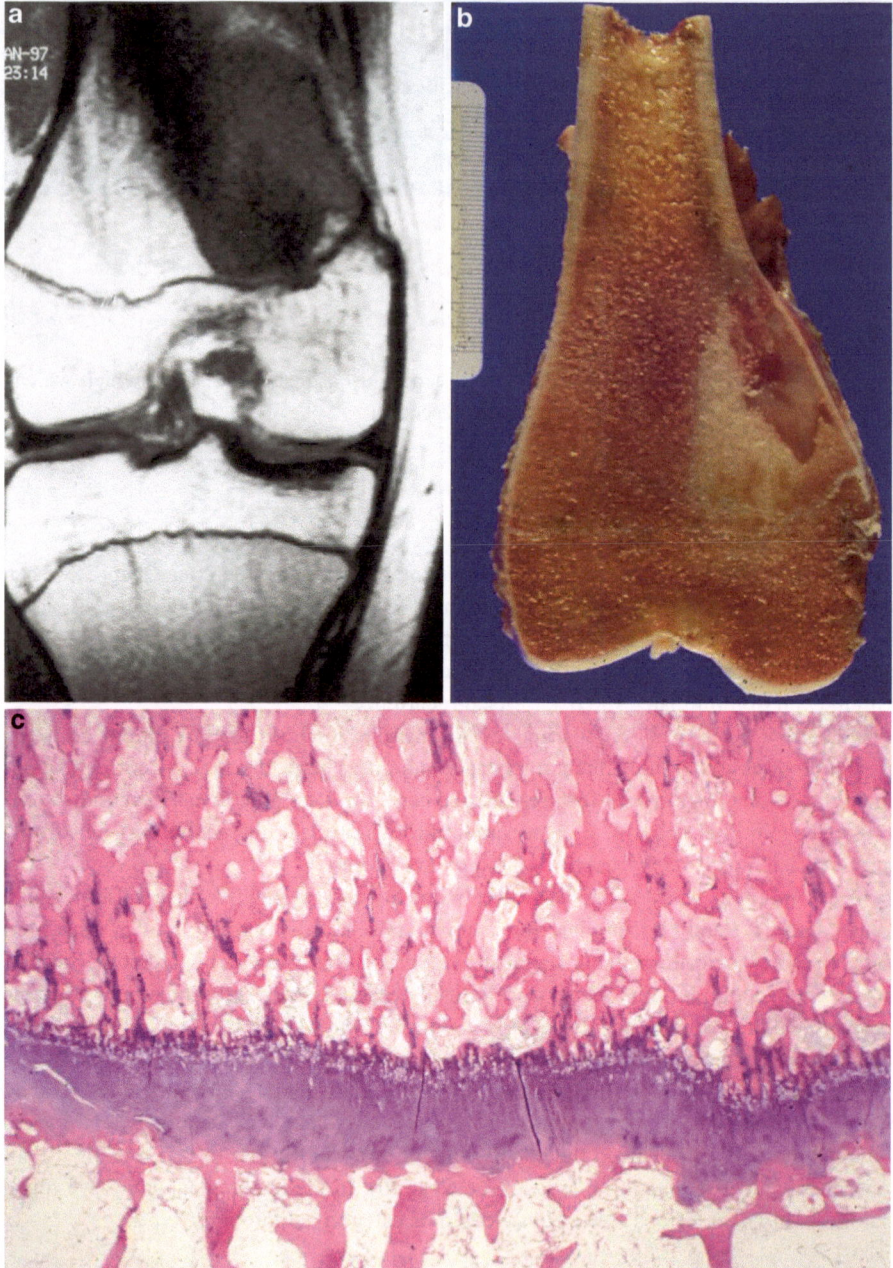

Fig. 7.1 (**a**) Osteosarcoma in the distal metaphysis of the femur of a 15-year-old boy. The tumour seems to cross the physis in the MRI image. (**b**, **c**) However, the histological study found no tumour cells crossing the physis

- The growth plate was not in contact with tumoural tissue.
- Areas of the growth plate were in contact with tumour tissue but were not penetrated by the tumour. Voluminous capillary sinusoids had introduced themselves between the columns of the matrix of the cartilage. The remainder of the physis appeared to be free of alterations.
- The physis was completely pierced by tumour tissue. The areas crossed by tumour were surrounded by zones of thinned cartilage, similar to what was observed in the second type of lesion.

The implication of these observations is that invasion of the epiphysis by the tumour progresses in a predictable manner: first there is a hypervascularisation reaction which leads to an early ossification of the growth plate, and after that the tumour crosses the physis.

The surgical treatment we recommend for these tumours depends on the stage of invasion of the epiphysis as revealed by MRI. The three possibilities are presented below.

1. *The tumour has crossed the physis*. In such cases, the preservation of the epiphysis is not possible (Fig. 7.2).

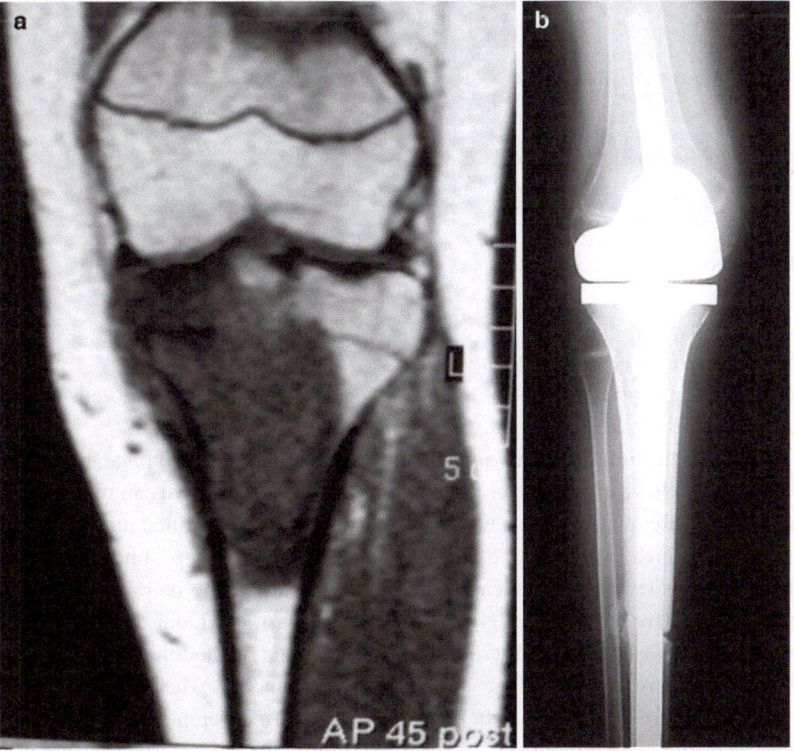

Fig. 7.2 (**a**) The growth plate has been crossed by this osteosarcoma in the proximal metaphysis of the tibia. (**b**) Reconstruction with a composite allograft-prosthesis

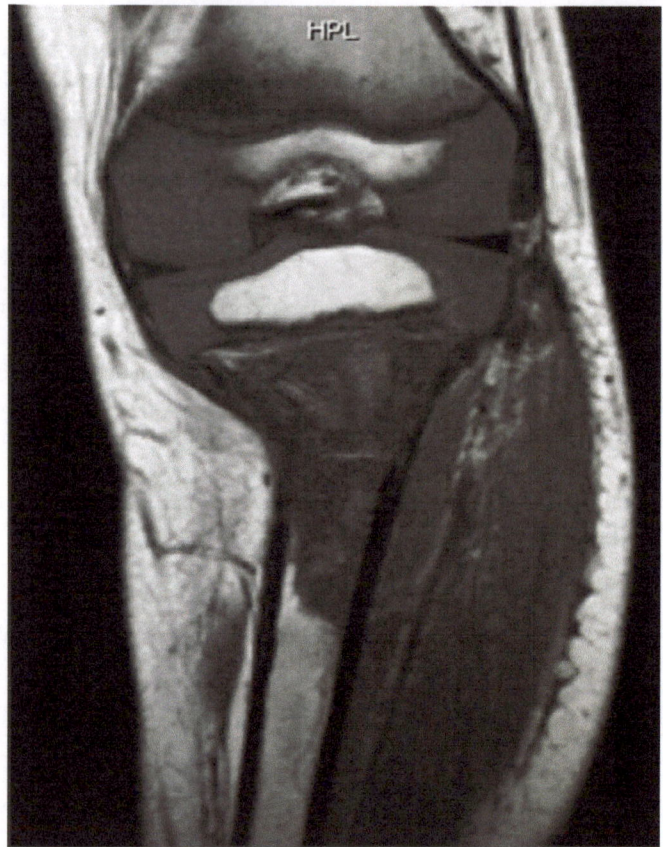

Fig. 7.3 Osteosarcoma in contact with the whole of the physis

2. *The tumour is in contact with the physis.*
- If all of the physis is affected (Fig. 7.3), the probability that tumour cells have crossed over the physis is very high (*see* Chap. 5).
- However, if the tumour is only in contact with part of the growth plate, tumour cells are less likely to have crossed over the physis and consequently we can try to preserve the epiphysis. After resection, the external fixation can be maintained until the appropriate manner in which to complete the surgical treatment (*see* Chap 8) has been decided on the basis of whether histological studies find tumour cells to be present in the physeal margin of the resection (Fig. 7.4). Before the advent of MRI, due to the lower accuracy of the other imaging methods employed, we used this methodology more frequently.
- An alternative method for preserving the epiphysis in cases when a tumour is in contact with only a part of the physis but does not cross it is intra-epiphyseal osteotomy, which may be useful especially in certain cases in children who are nearing the end of growth.
3. *The tumour is near but not in contact with the physis.* Physeal distraction before excision is, in our experience, the best technique in such cases (Fig. 7.5). The safety of

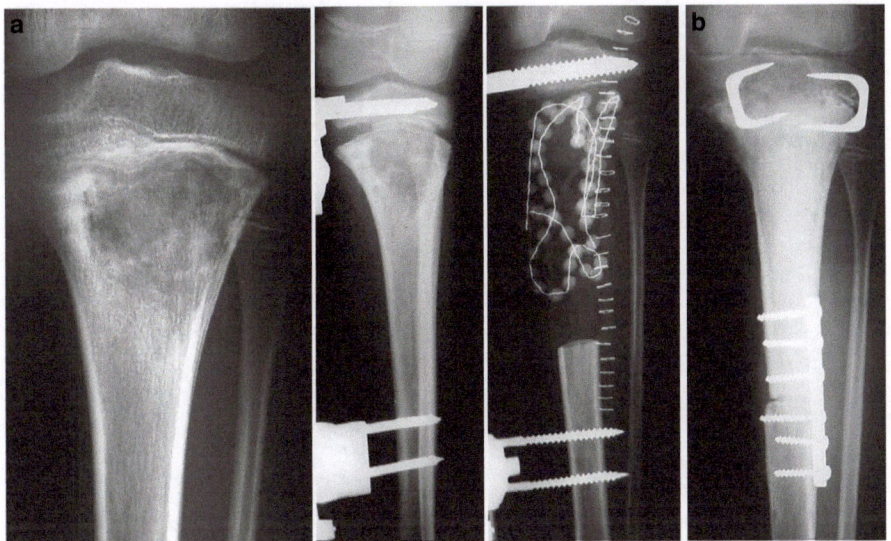

Fig. 7.4 Physeal distraction according to Cañadell's technique in a case in which involvement of the physis was uncertain, before the MRI era. (**a**) External fixation was kept in place after resection until histological study of the resection margins had been carried out. (**b**) After histological confirmation of the absence of tumour cells in the metaphyseal margin of the resection, the reconstruction was carried out with an intercalary allograft

physeal distraction and the fact that it can preserve the whole epiphysis and most of the growth plate make it superior to other techniques such as epiphyseal osteotomy.

The fact that there are no anastomoses between epiphyseal and metaphyseal vessels, the possibility of using imaging methods to determine whether or not the tumour has involved the epiphysis, and the Cañadell technique for resection through physeal distraction[1,11] together make it feasible, in selected cases, to preserve the epiphysis and the joint during tumour resection.

Physeal distraction was used only in tumours of the distal femur, proximal tibia, distal tibia, and distal fibula. In locations such as the proximal fibula or proximal femur, physeal distraction was not used for obvious reasons (Fig. 7.6).

In tumours involving the proximal metaphysis of the humerus, the particular morphology of the growth plate makes it possible to employ physeal distraction (Fig. 7.7).

The presence of a pathological fracture (Fig. 7.8) contraindicates physeal distraction because the distraction will occur through the fracture instead of through the growth plate.

In such cases, intra-epiphyseal osteotomy could be used to conserve the epiphysis. However, if fracture heals during neo-adjuvant chemotherapy period, it is still possible to perform physeal distraction (Fig. 7.9).

Finally, note that physeal distraction serves no purpose in cases of diaphyseal tumours with a safe margin between the tumour and the physis[5] (Fig. 7.10).

7

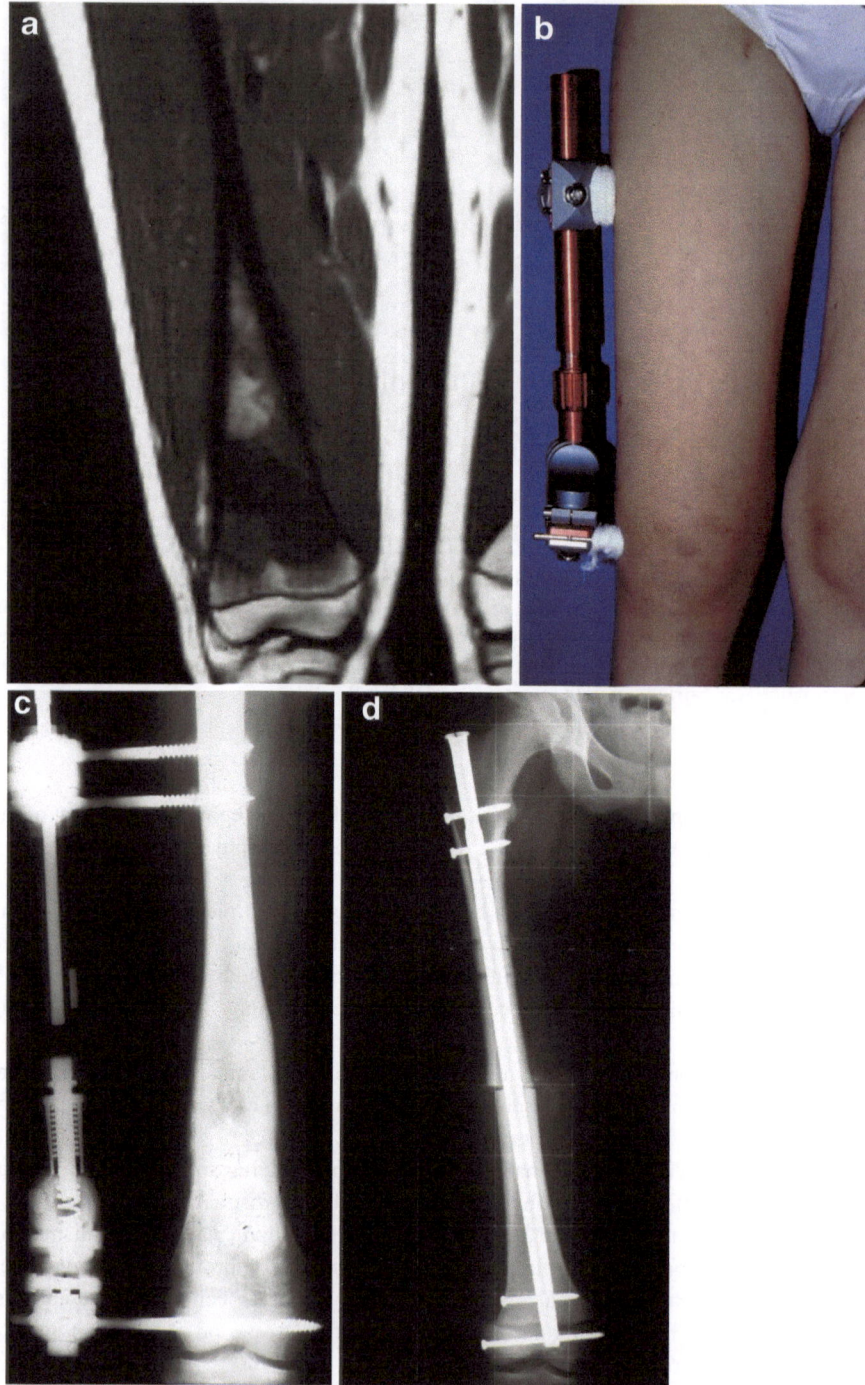

Fig. 7.5 (**a**) Osteosarcoma in the distal femur. The tumour is not in contact with the growth plate. There are some areas of oedema between the tumour and the physis. (**b**, **c**) Physeal distraction was performed. (**d**) Reconstruction was by intercalary allograft

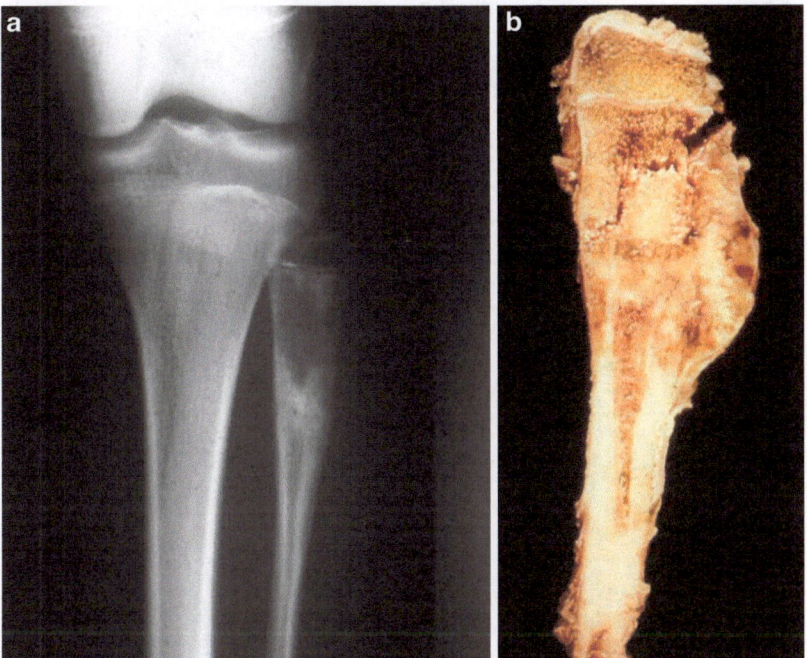

Fig. 7.6 Osteosarcoma in the proximal metaphysis of the fibula of a 15-year-old girl. In such cases, it would not be appropriate to attempt to use physeal distraction and to preserve the epiphysis because of the risk of lesion to the peroneal nerve when placing the pins. Aside from this consideration, in this patient, the loss of the epiphysis does not imply any impairment in knee function

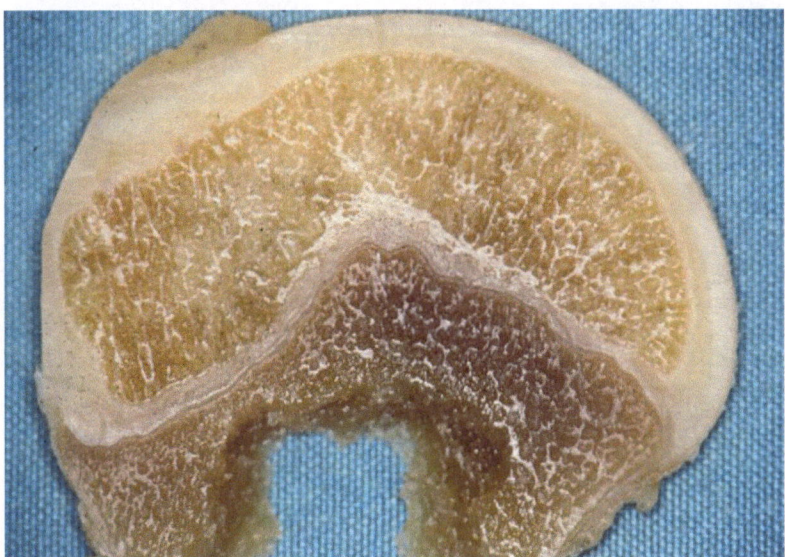

Fig. 7.7 The particular morphology of the growth plate of the proximal humerus allows placement of pins for physeal distraction

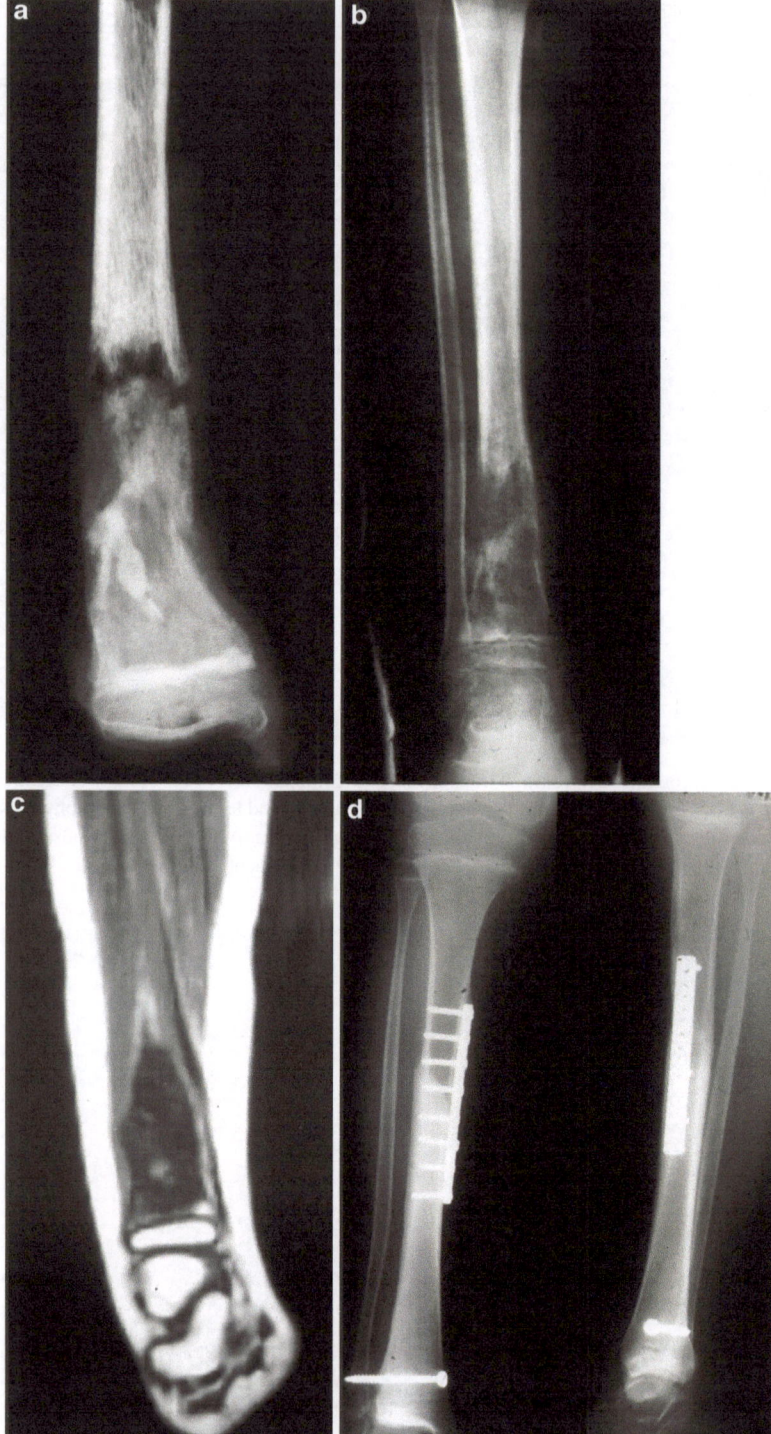

Fig. 7.8 (a) Pathological fracture in the distal tibia of a 9-year-old boy affected by an osteosarcoma. (b) The tumour did not transgress the physis. (c) X-ray of the resected piece. (d) Reconstruction was done by osteoarticular allograft

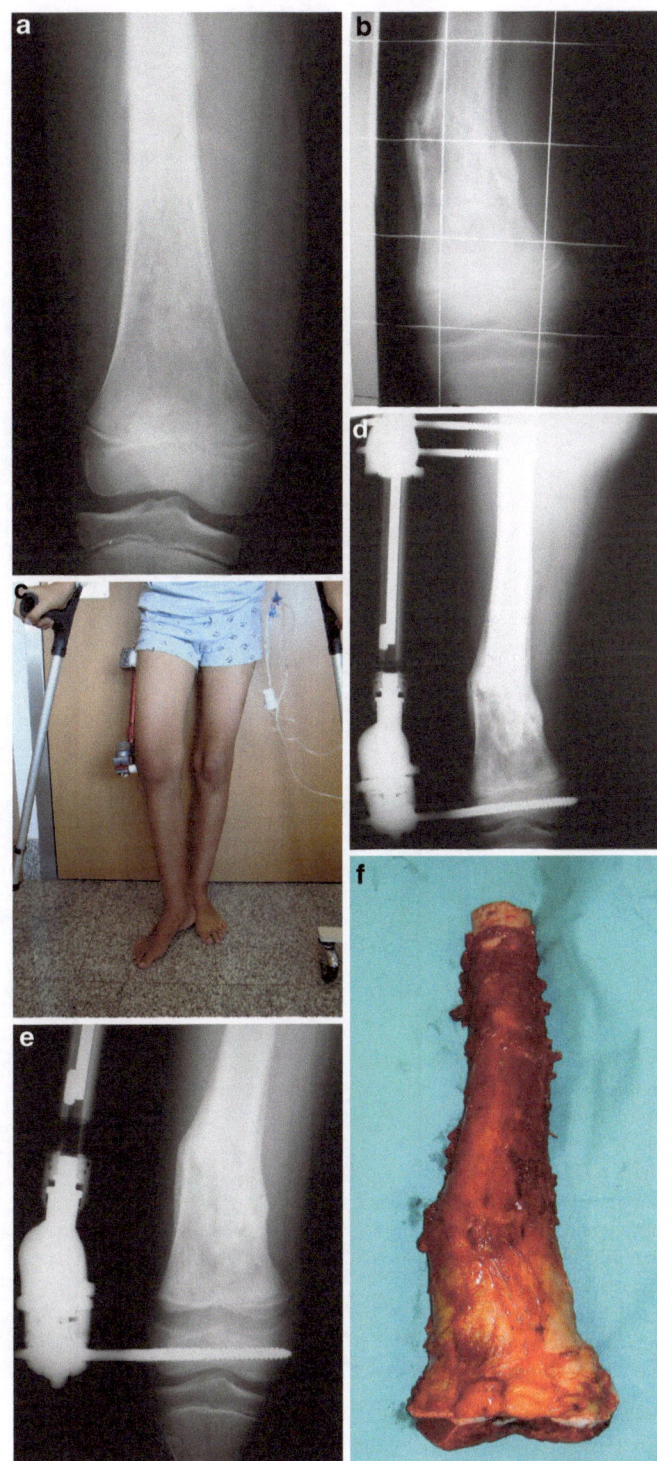

Fig. 7.9 (**a**) Ewing's sarcoma in the distal femur of a 10-year-old boy. Note the ostelysis in the metaphysis and the Codman triangle in the middle shaft. (**b**) Few days after diagnosis, this patient suffered a pathological fracture which healed after a few weeks. (**c**) The external fixation was placed. (**d**) Note the varus and shortening due to the fracture. (**e**) Epiphysiolysis was successful (**f**) resected pieze. Note a fine layer of growth plate tissue covering the distal margin of resection

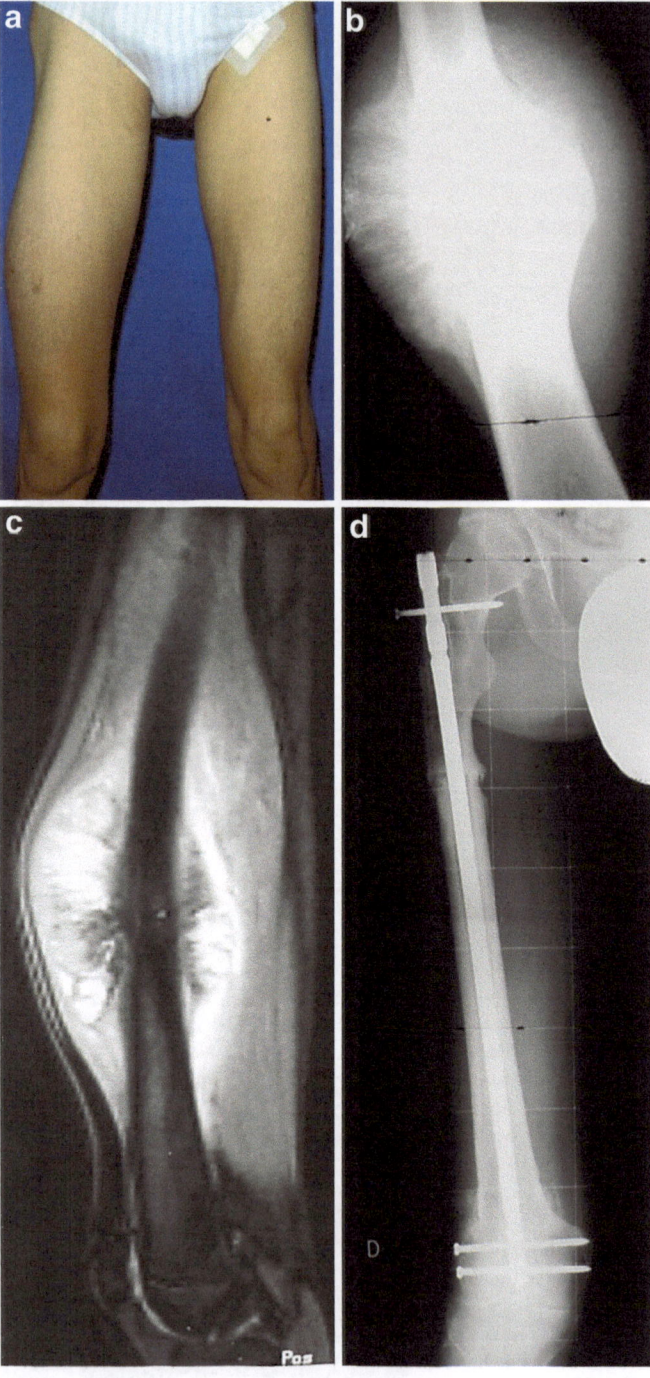

Fig. 7.10 Clinical picture (**a**) and X-ray (**b**) of an osteosarcoma in a 15-year-old boy. There was a safe margin between the tumour and the growth plate (**c**). The tumour was resected and reconstruction was carried out with an intercalary allograft (**d**)

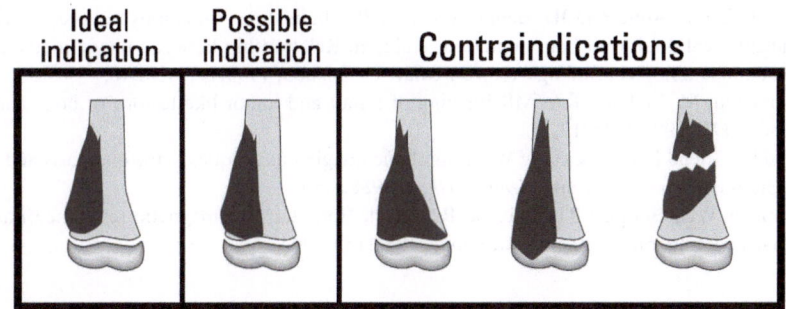

Fig. 7.11 MRI-based indications and contraindications for physeal distraction before resection of metaphyseal tumours

A summary of the MRI-based indications and contraindications for tumour resection with physeal distraction in order to preserve the epiphysis is given in Fig. 7.11.

Of the patients we have operated on in accordance with the Cañadell technique, none have suffered a local recurrence of the tumour in the retaicned epiphysis.

References

1. Cañadell J, Forriol F, Cara JA, San-Julian M. Removal of metaphyseal bone tumors with preservation of the epiphysis. Physeal distraction before excision. In: Cañadell J, San-Julian M, Cara JA, eds. *Surgical Treatment of Malignant Bone Tumors*. Pamplona: Ediciones Universidad de Navarra; 1995: 153–160.
2. De Pablos J, Cañadell J, Vazquez J, Idoate, M. Clinical study on the barrier effect of the physis in metaphyseal osteosarcoma. In: Cañadell J, Sierrasesúmaga L, Calvo F, Ganoza C, eds. *Treatment of Malignant Bone Tumors in Children and Adolescents*. Pamplona: Ediciones Universidad de Navarra; 1991:221–245.
3. Exner GU, Von Hochstetter AR, Augustiny N, Von Schulthess G. Magnetic resonance imaging in malignant bone tumors. *Int Orthop*. 1990;14:49.
4. Golfieri R, Baddeley H, Pringle JS, Souhami R. The role of the STIR sequence in magnetic resonance imaging examination of bone tumors. *Br J Radiol*. 1990;63:251.
5. Grimer RJ, Bielack S, Flege S, et al. and from The European Musculo Skeletal Oncology Society (EMSOS) Periosteal osteosarcoma. A European review of outcome. *Eur J Cancer*. 2005 Dec;41(18):2806–2811.
6. Hudson TM, Hamlin DS, Ennekingg WF, Peterson H. Magnetic resonance imaging of bone and soft tissue tumors. *Skeletal Radiol*. 1985;13:134.
7. Kattapuram SV. Imaging of musculoskeletal tumors. *Current Opin Orthopaed*. 1991;2:781.
8. Knop J, Delling G, Heise U, Winkler K. Scintigraphic of tumor regression during preoperative chemotherapy of osteosarcoma: correlation of Tc-99m-methylene diphosphonate parametric imaging with surgical histopathology. Skeletal Radiol. 1990;19:165.
9. Lemmi MA, Fletcher RB, Marina NM, et al. Use of LMR imaging to assess results of chemotherapy for Ewing sarcoma. *AJR*. 1990;155:343.
10. O'Flanagan SJ, Stack JP, Mccee HM, Dervan P, Hurson B. Imaging of intramedullary tumor spread in osteosarcoma: a comparison of techniques. *J Bone Joint Surg (Am)*. 1991; 73-A:998–1001.

11. San Julian M, Aquerreta JD, Benito A, Cañadell J. Indications for epiphyseal preservation in metaphyseal malignant bone tumors of children. Relationship between image methods and anatomopathological findings". *Am J Pediatr Orthopaed*. 1999;19:543–548.
12. Sundaram M, McLeod RA. MR imaging of tumor and tumor-like lesions of bone and soft tissue. *AJR*. 1990;155:817.
13. Vander Griend RA, Ennekingg WF. Radiologic imaging techniques in the diagnosis and treatment of osteogenic sarcoma. *Semin Orthop*. 1988;3:59.
14. Zimmer WD, Berquist TH, Mcleod RA, et al. Bone tumors: magnetic resonance imaging versus computer tomography. *Radiology*. 1985;155:709.

Conservation of the Epiphysis While Removing Metaphyseal Bone Tumours: Epiphysiolysis Before Excision

8

José Cañadell, Mikel San-Julian, Jose A. Cara, and Francisco Forriol

Abstract Physeal distraction, not for lengthening but for epiphysiolysis, provides a safe margin of resection in selected cases. The technique does not delay tumour treatment: all that is required is 15 min, a fortnight before the established date for surgery, for placing the external fixator.

Introduction

Physeal distraction has been extensively used for bone lengthening[4-6] and for correcting angular deformities.[1,2,8] We now describe its use in facilitating the excision of malignant bone tumours of the metaphysis while preserving the epiphysis.

The absence of anastomoses between epiphyseal and metaphyseal vessels means that in those cases where imaging methods determine that the epiphysis has not been affected by the tumour, it is possible to conserve the epiphysis and the joint while resecting the tumour. This is made possible by physeal distraction according to Cañadell's technique.

Patients and Methods

Between July 1980 and December 2007, we operated on more than 800 patients with paediatric bone sarcomas. One hundred thirty six patients received intercalary reconstructions, many by means of physeal distraction. Of these 136, the mean age was 9.4 years; there were similar numbers of males and females. The histological diagnosis was osteosarcoma in two-thirds of the patients and Ewing's sarcoma in the remaining one-third.

José Cañadell (✉)
Department of Orthopedic Surgery, University of Navarra, Avda Pio XII s/n,
31008 Pamplona, Spain
e-mail: mmlopez@unav.es

J. Cañadell and M. San-Julian (eds.), *Pediatric Bone Sarcomas: Epiphysiolysis Before Excision*,
DOI: 10.1007/978-1-84882-130-9_8, © Springer-Verlag London Limited 2011

The indications for Cañadell's technique were:

1. *Location of the tumour in the metaphyseal region.*
2. *The physeal cartilage had to be open.* A patient's age is an important consideration here. In about half of our paediatric patients, the tumour had not involved the physis; the mean age of this group was 11 years. In patients who have nearly finished growing, the probability of tumoural cells having crossed the physis is higher, and it is more difficult to achieve physeal distraction. Other authors[7] have reported a similar incidence of micro- or gross extension to the epiphysis from metaphyseal bone tumours.
3. *The tumour must not have transgressed the physis.* Radiography, arteriography, CT, and particularly MRI were used to demonstrate this pre-operatively, and histological examination was used to corroborate this.[3]

Operative Technique

The surgical technique usually consists of two phases:

Phase one (Fig. 8.1). Two pins are inserted into the epiphysis and another two into the diaphysis 8–10 cm away from the tumour. An external monolateral fixator with a T-shaped piece (Fig. 8.2) for the epiphyseal pins is attached (Fig. 8.3). We usually use Schanz pins of 5 or 6 mm diameter. In very young children, 4 mm pins could be strong enough for achieving epiphysiolysis.

Distraction is begun in the operating room and continues at the rate of 1–1.5 mm/day until 1 or 2 cm of distraction is achieved. During the first few days nothing happens, but

First surgical step   10-15 days

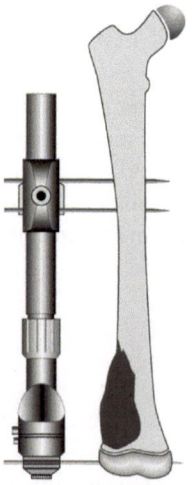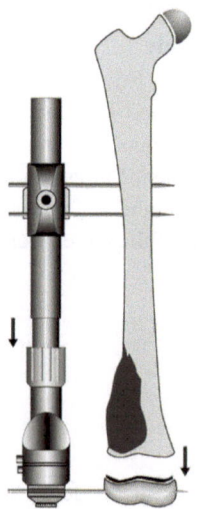

Fig. 8.1 Diagram showing the first surgical step

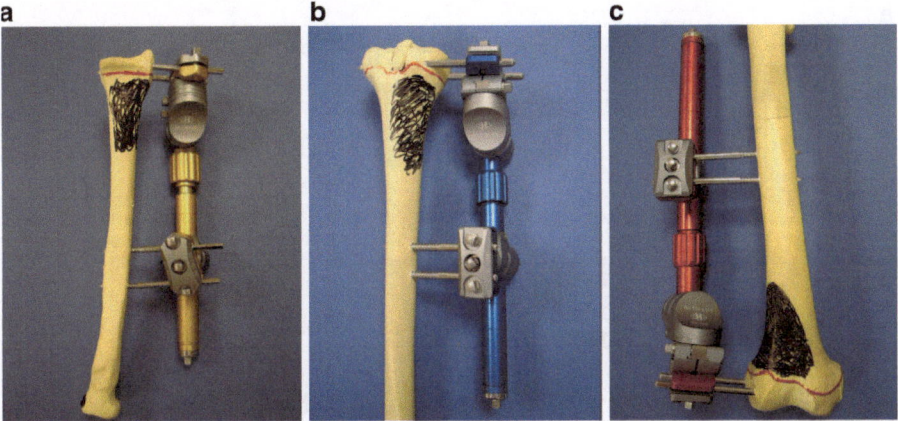

Fig. 8.2 (**a–c**) Devices used in young children for distal tibia, distal fibula, and distal radius (yellow) and in adolescents for proximal tibia and humerus (blue) and distal femur (red). All devices have a T-shaped piece in order to put the two epiphyseal pins perpendicular to the diaphysis

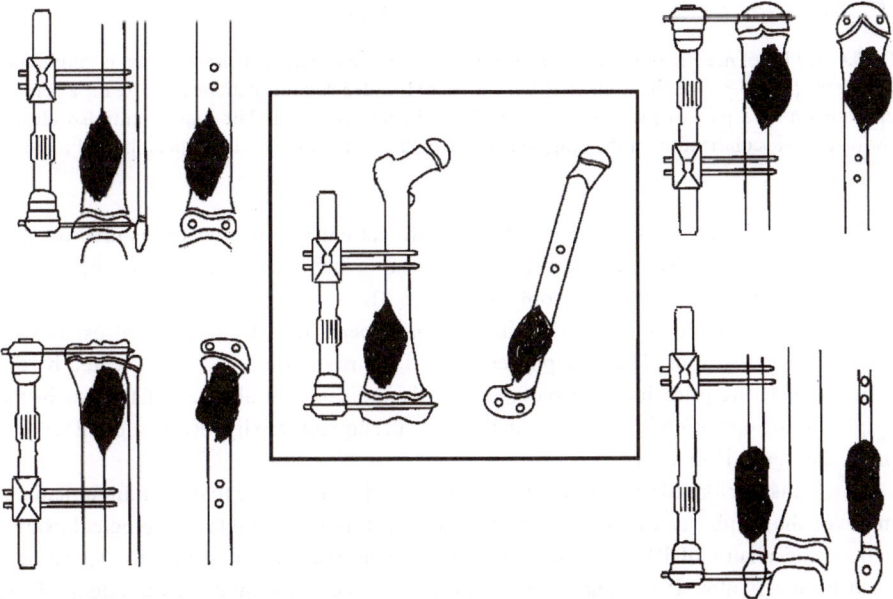

Fig. 8.3 Diagrams showing the placement of the pins in distal femur, proximal and distal tibia, proximal humerus, and distal fibula

usually after between 7 and 14 days of distraction, the patient refers pain indicating rupture of the growth plate: radiography will show disruption of the physis. In our series of 136 patients, the mean time over which distraction was applied was 10 days.

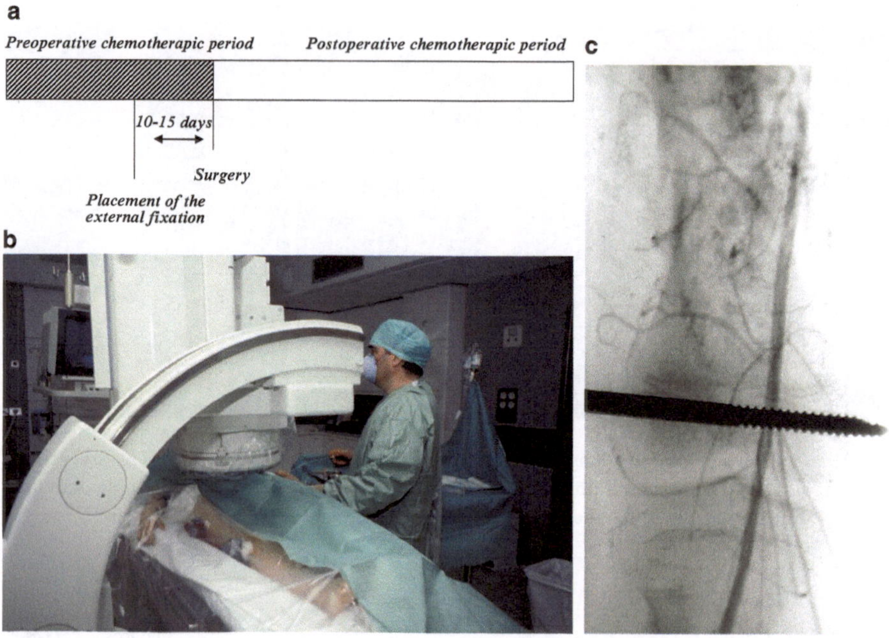

a

Preoperative chemotherapic period   Postoperative chemotherapic period   **c**

10-15 days

Surgery

Placement of the
external fixation

b

Fig. 8.4 (**a**) It not necessary to delay the protocol of treatment. The first surgical step is carried out during the pre-operative chemotherapy period. (**b, c**) In osteosarcoma patients, we use intra-arterial cisplatinum as a part of the neo-adjuvant chemotherapy protocol. The angiogram also clearly shows that vascularization of the epiphysis is not connected with that of the metaphyseal tumour

This first phase can be carried out while the patient is finishing the course of neo-adjuvant chemotherapy. Despite the external fixator being in place, even intra-arterial procedures can be used without problems[9] (Fig. 8.4).

Phase two. En-bloc resection of the tumour is performed by diaphyseal osteotomy, leaving a wide margin. The metaphyseal end of the resection is already effected by the distraction. If the prior imaging methods clearly indicated an absence of tumour in the epiphysis, the operation is completed in this second surgical step by reconstruction with an intercalary graft (Fig. 8.5).

In the past, before MRI, with cases where we could not be sure that the tumour had not involved the epiphysis, the resected tumour was sent immediately for histological examination, and chains of PMMA containing gentamycin were inserted into the space held open by the fixator. If the pathologist reported absence of tumour at the edges of the resected segment, the chains of beads were withdrawn and a bone graft was inserted (*see also* Fig. 7.4). If, on the other hand, the pathologist were to find tumour cells, the procedure would be to resect the epiphysis and reconstruct the limb by other means: prosthesis, osteoarticular allograft, or arthrodesis. This was only necessary in one patient, whose prosthetic reconstruction proceeded without problem, and who suffered no local recurrence. MRI has removed the uncertainty over epiphysis involvement, and with it the need for this "three-step variant" of the technique (Figs. 8.6 and 8.7).

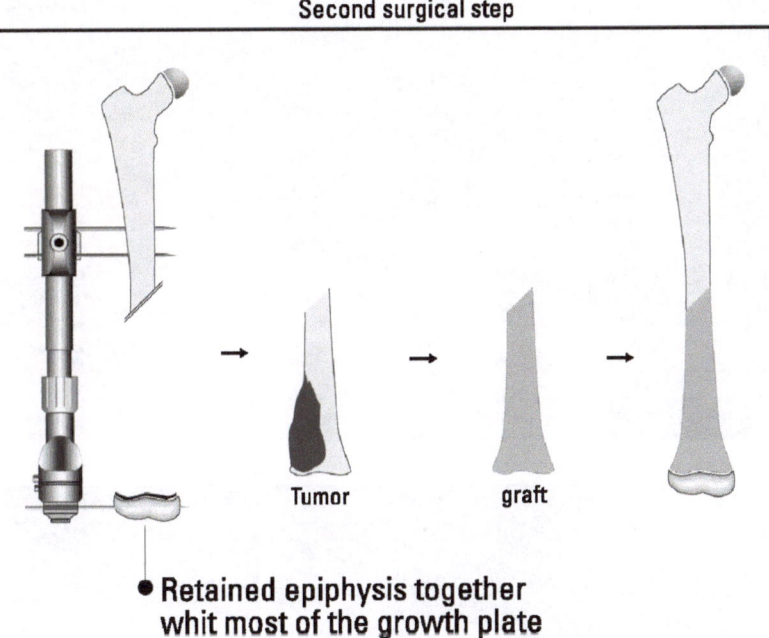

Second surgical step

Tumor   graft

• Retained epiphysis together
  whit most of the growth plate

Fig. 8.5 Diagram showing resection and reconstruction

The choice of the kind of osteosynthesis device in the graft and in the remaining physis and epiphysis can play an important role in the final leg-length discrepancy (*see* Chap. 9). In this respect, for children near the end of growth, it may be appropriate to insert an allograft longer than the resected piece.

Discussion

When resecting a tumour, the surgeon must be certain that no malignant tissue is left behind. Many authors agree that a 3–5 cm margin is safe in bone sarcomas. This means that, when the tumour is in the metaphysis, resection requires the loss of the adjacent joint. However, by definition, the wide margin is taken to be of a layer of normal tissue, as opposed to reactive or inflammatory tissues, surrounding the tumour. Thus, a safe margin in the context of a metaphyseal tumour could be obtained without sacrificing the epiphysis. In tumours that do not cross the growth plate, our technique, using previous physeal distraction, provides a safe margin while averting loss of the epiphysis. We believe that, when present, the growth cartilage itself provides a dependable margin of safety and that the 3–5 cm margin suggested by most authors is unnecessary. This view is supported by the fact that in our series no tumour recurred locally in the retained epiphysis.

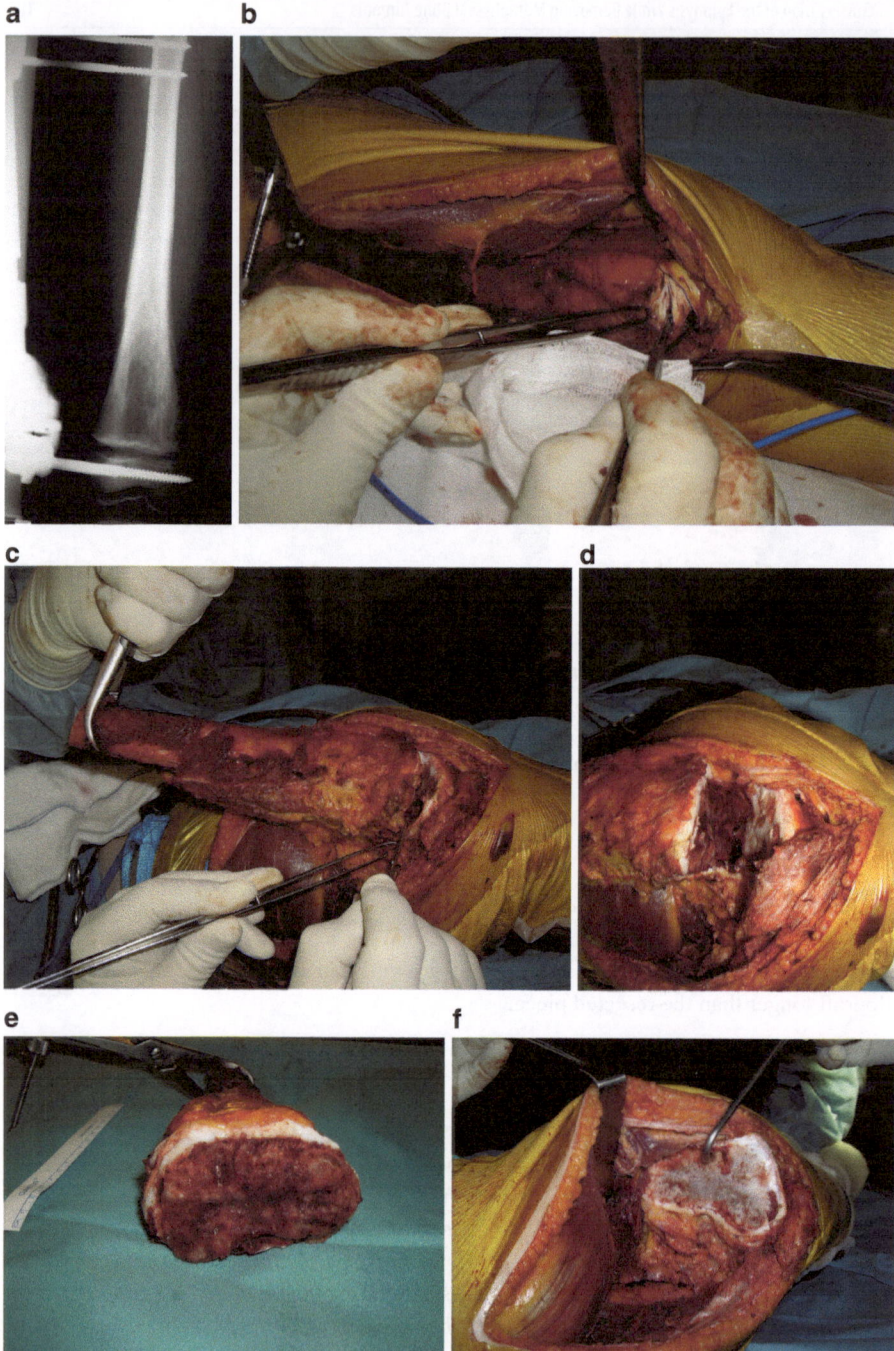

Fig. 8.6 After distraction (**a**), surgery is easier. The perichondrium is cut (**b–d**). We only need a diaphyseal osteotomy (**c**), because the metaphyseal "osteotomy" is already done. The resected piece is covered by a thin layer of growth plate which constitutes a safe margin (**e**), while most of the growth plate remains attached to the epiphysis in the patient (**f**)

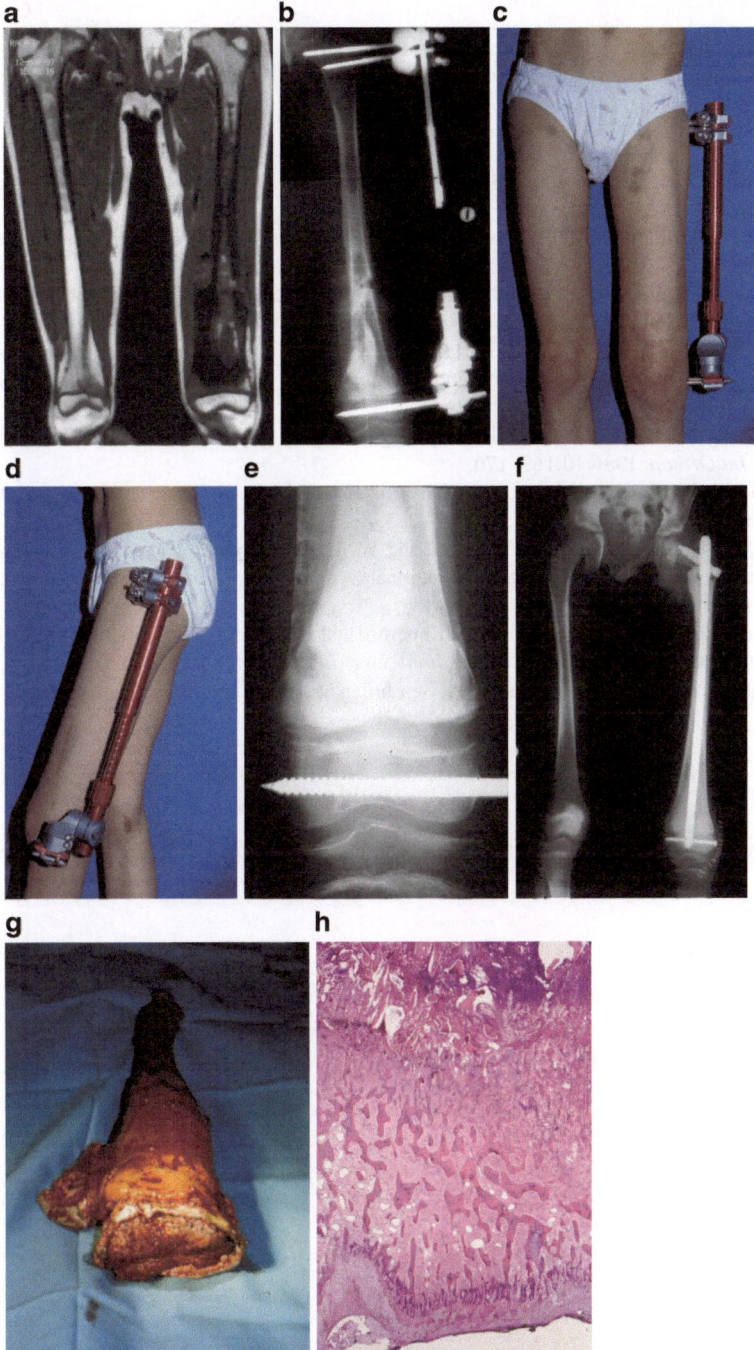

Fig. 8.7 Osteosarcoma involving two-thirds of the femur in a 13-year-old boy. MRI (**a**) shows some oedema between the tumour and the growth plate. In this case, the proximal pins were placed in the femoral neck due to the tumoural extension (**b–d**). Physeal distraction was achieved (**e**). Reconstruction was carried out with an intercalary allograft in the second surgical step (**f**). The allograft used was 2 cm longer than the resected piece (**g**, **h**). The resected piece (**g**) together with the biopsy scar. Staining of the distal margin with Indian ink (**h**) shows that the margin is free of tumour, because there is a thin layer of growth plate cells covering the resected bone

References

1. Cañadell J, De Pablos J. Breaking bone bridges by physeal distraction: a new approach. *Int Orthop*. 1985;9:223–229.
2. Cañadell J, De Pablos J. Correction of angular deformities by physeal distraction. *Clin Orthop*. 1992;283:98.
3. Daffner RH, Lupetin AR, Dash N, et al. MRI in the detection of malignant infiltration of bone marrow. *AJR*. 1986;146:353–358.
4. De Bastiani G, Aldegheri R, Renzi Brivio L, Triviella G. Limb lengthening by distraction of the epiphyseal plate. A comparison of two techniques in the rabbit. *J Bone Joint Surg (Br)*. 1986; 68-B:545–549.
5. De Pablos J, Villas C, Cañadell J. Bone lengthening by physeal distraction: an experimental study. *Int Orthop*. 1986;10:163–170.
6. Monticelli G, Spinelli R. Distraction epiphysiolysis as a method of limb lengthening. III Clinical applications. *Clin Orthop*. 1991;154:274–285.
7. Neel M, Bush C, Scarborough M, Enneking W. Transepiphyseal extension of osteosarcoma. Abstract book of the 8th ISOLS (International Symposium on Limb Salvage, Florence, May 10th–12th, 1995; pp. 107.
8. Peltonen JI, Karaharku EO, Alitalo I. Experimental epiphysiolysis distraction producing and correcting angular deformities. *J Bone Joint Surg (Br)*. 1984;66-B:598–602.
9. Sierrasesúmaga L, Antillon F, Patiño A, San Julian M. *Oncología Pediátrica*. Madrid: Pearson; 2005.

Mikel San-Julian and José Cañadell

Abstract There were no local recurrences in the retained epiphysis. The rate of complications was similar to that with other reconstruction procedures. The retained growth plate can continue growing. Functional results are excellent.

Control of Disease

Patients were treated according to the protocol of treatment for osteosarcoma and Ewing's sarcoma at the University Clinic of Navarra.[34,35] Mean follow-up was 124 months (range of 12–288 months), and most patients were followed up for at least 2 years. There were no cases of local recurrence in the epiphyseal region, and only one in the diaphysis, which occurred 22 months after the operation. At present, the disease-free survival rate is 85%. This rate is slightly better than that for the overall series of osteosarcoma and Ewing's sarcoma patients (Fig. 9.1); tumours that did not cross the physis may have been less aggressive than those that did. Other authors, reporting on surgery without preservation of the epiphysis,[26] present similar results (85% of survival).[19]

Histological Study of Margins

Previous studies by our team indicate that invasion of the epiphysis by a tumour seems to be a question of time: there is a hypervascularization reaction which leads to an early ossification of the growth plate, and after that, the tumour transgresses the physis. However, for epiphysiolysis to be indicated, the tumour must not have crossed the physis. For the series of patients reported here, imaging methods were able to predict whether the physis had been involved by the tumour.

Histological examination of resected pieces confirmed in all cases that the tumour had not involved the growth plate. We used Indian ink staining to study the physeal margin of

Mikel San-Julian (✉)
Department of Orthopedic Surgery, University Clinic of Navarra, Avda. Pio XII, s/n,
Pamplona, Navarra 31008, Spain
e-mail: msjulian@unav.es

J. Cañadell and M. San-Julian (eds.), *Pediatric Bone Sarcomas: Epiphysiolysis Before Excision*,
DOI: 10.1007/978-1-84882-130-9_9, © Springer-Verlag London Limited 2011

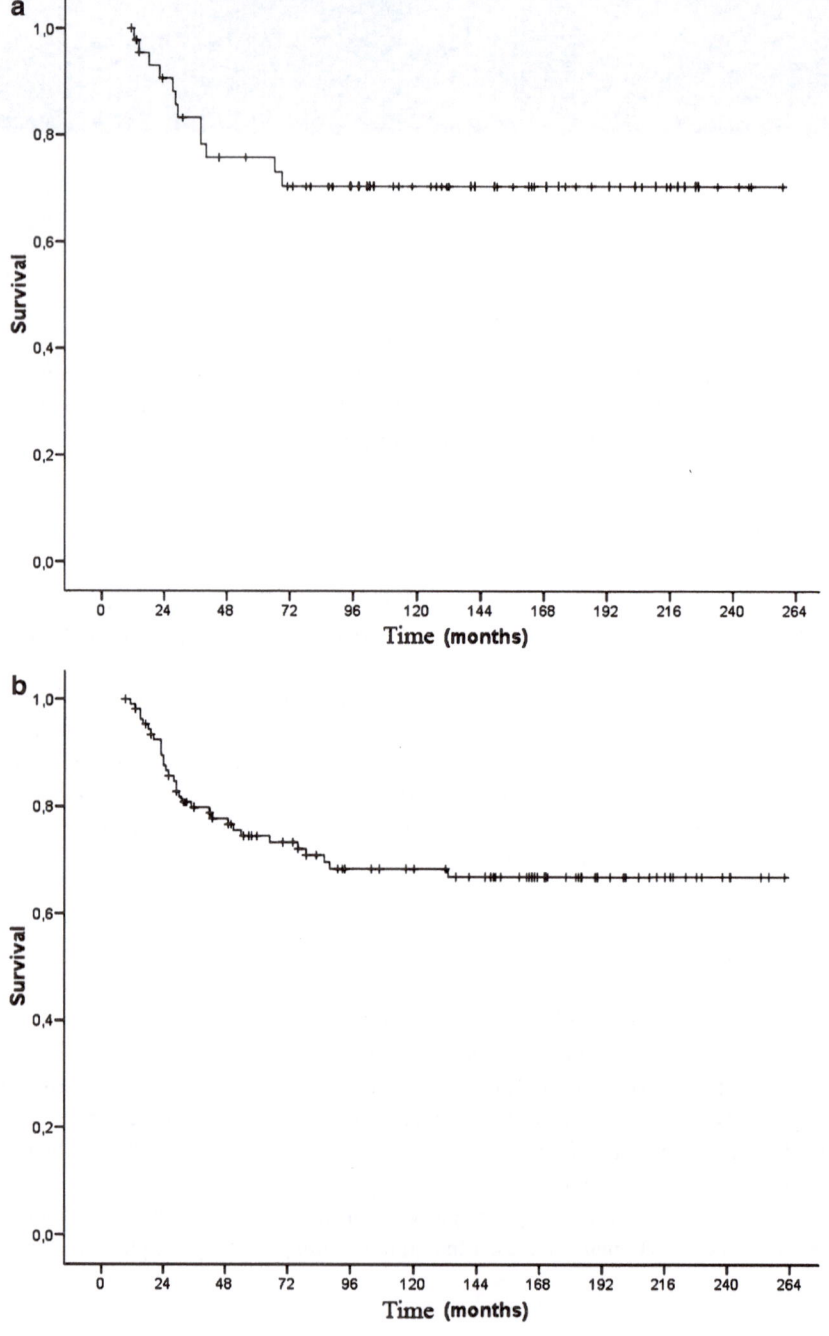

Fig. 9.1 Long-term survival of osteosarcoma (**a**) and Ewing's sarcoma patients (**b**) treated at our institution. DFS at 15 years is 72% in osteosarcoma and 68% in Ewing's sarcoma

resection, where, because at the rate of distraction employed (1 mm/day) the growth plate is disrupted at the degenerative layer of cells, there is a thin layer of growth plate cells covering the bone (Fig. 9.2). The rate of distraction has also the result that most of the growth plate is retained with the epiphysis.

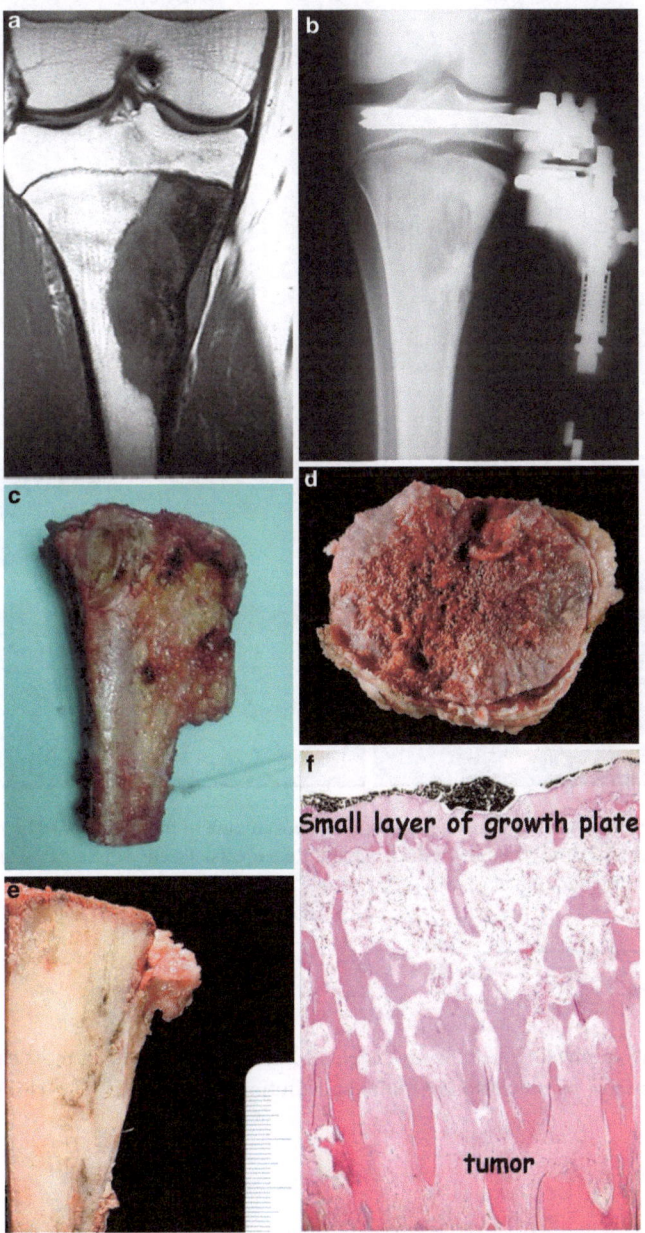

Fig. 9.2 (**a**) Proximal tibia osteosarcoma apparently in contact with the growth plate. (**b**) After epi-physiolysis. (**c-f**) This is, by definition, a wide margin. (**f**) Indian ink shows the margin is free of tumor

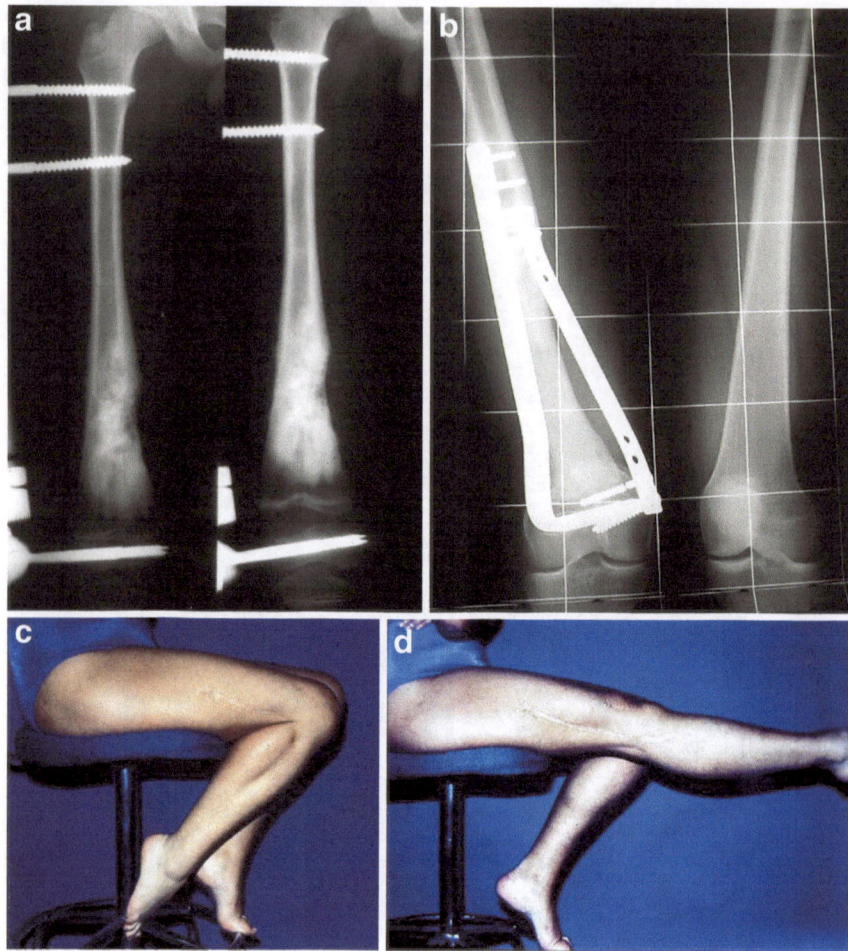

Fig. 9.3 (**a**) Physeal distraction in a metaphyseal osteosarcoma of the femur. (**b**) The reconstruction was carried out with autografts from the tibia and iliac crests. Twenty-three years after operation, the joint (**b**) and the functional results (**c, d**) remain excellent

Limb Function

Preserving the epiphysis results in an excellent functional outcome in most cases. In addition, the long-term complications of joint substitution are avoided[2–4,27–29] (Figs. 9.2–9.6).

Complications

Infection. This occurred in 7% of patients, and the risk of infection is the same as in other limb salvage procedures. The risk is not higher because the external fixator is placed for

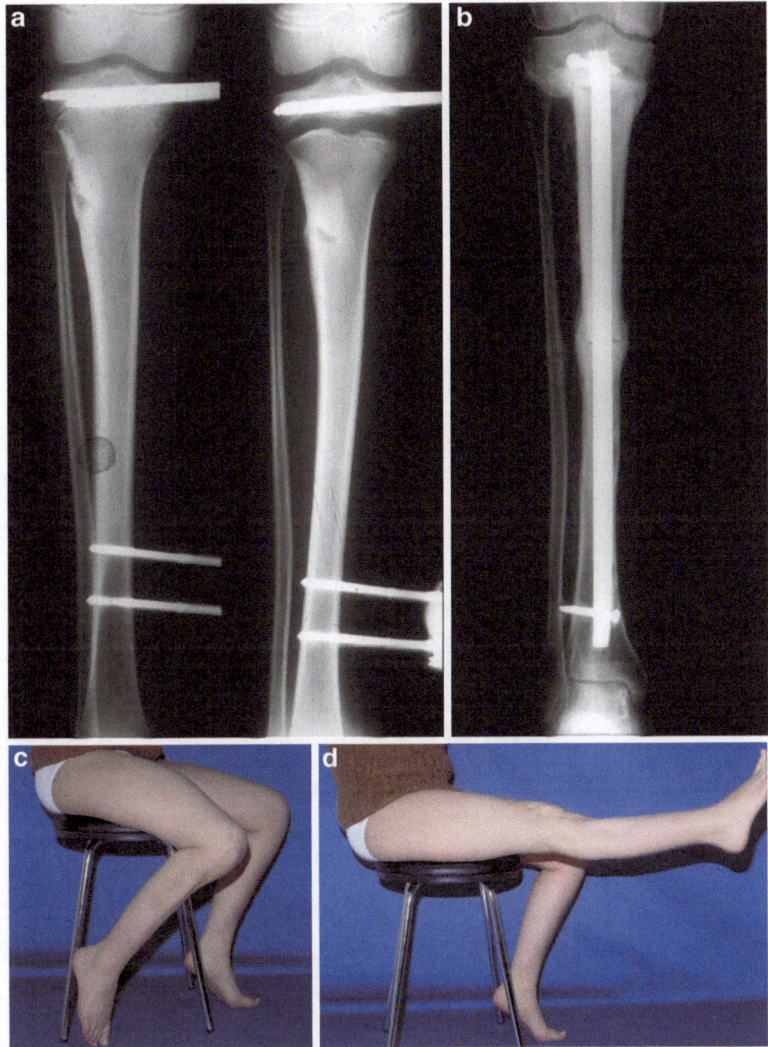

Fig. 9.4 (**a**) Ewing's sarcoma in the proximal metaphysis of the tibia. Physeal distraction was performed. (**b**) The reconstruction was carried out with an intercalary allograft. (**c, d**) Functional result

only 10–15 days (Fig. 9.7). Of the cases with infection, some were cured by systemic antibiotic therapy, but most required removal of an allograft, reattachment of the external fixator, insertion of gentamicin-impregnated cement, systemic antibiotic therapy,[7] and, after elimination of the infection, implantation of a new allograft. The risk of infection is higher in allografts in comparison to autografts. This is another reason for choosing autografts for reconstruction in young children or after resection of small tumours.

Non-union of the graft. About 14% of patients required a further operation, with the addition of autologous grafts, to achieve union between the allograft and the host bone. Healing was achieved in all cases.

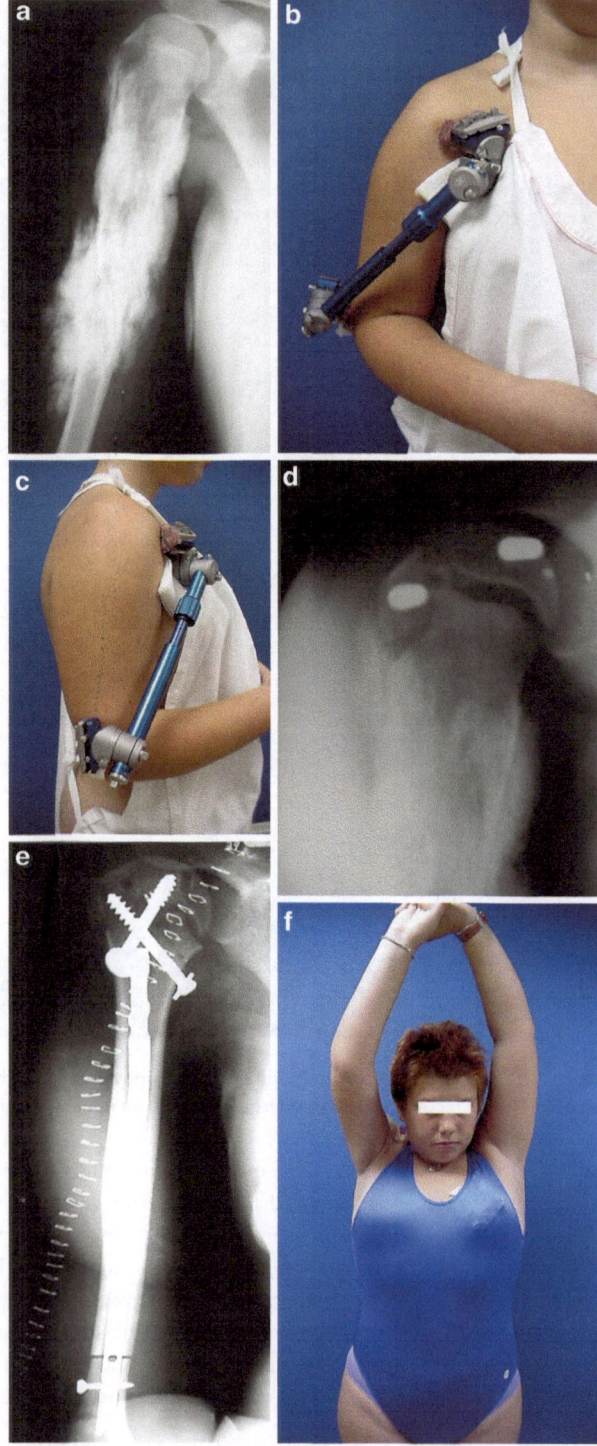

Fig. 9.5 (**a–c**) In the proximal humerus, due to the particular morphology of this growth plate, the pins should be placed anteriorly in the humeral head (*see also* Fig. 7.7) and posteriolaterally in the distal part, in order to avoid radial nerve damage. (**d**) After distraction, reconstruction was carried out (**e**) with an allograft. (**f**) Abduction of the shoulder is almost complete because the joint, the attachment of the rotator cuff, and the axillary nerve could be preserved

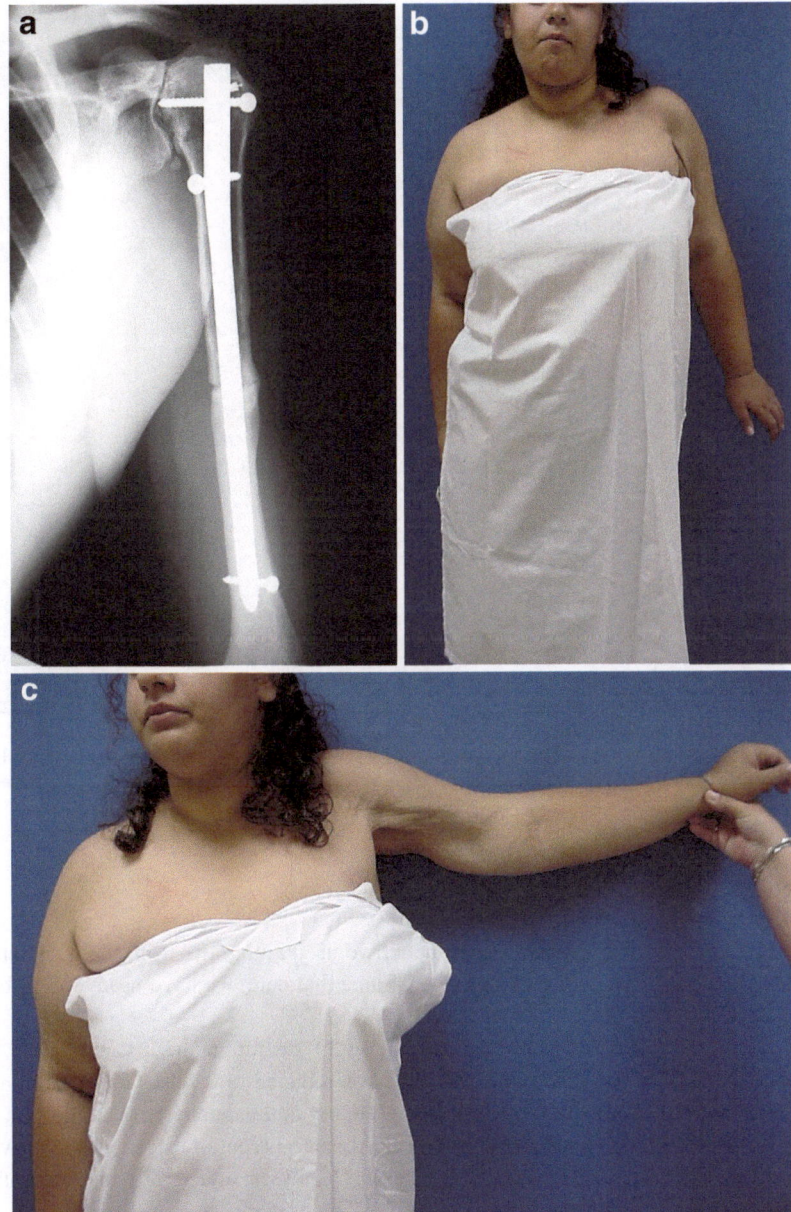

Fig. 9.6 (**a**) Osteoarticular allograft for reconstruction of the shoulder after resection of a Ewing's sarcoma in the proximal humerus. When the joint cannot be preserved, abduction of the shoulder, both active (**b**) and passive (**c**), is poor

Others. As with other tumoural resection procedures, peroneal nerve palsy can occur. Chemotherapy, because of its neurotoxicity, is also involved in this palsy. Another complication is fracture of the united allograft, which can usually be successfully treated by osteosynthesis with a plate and screws and autologous graft.

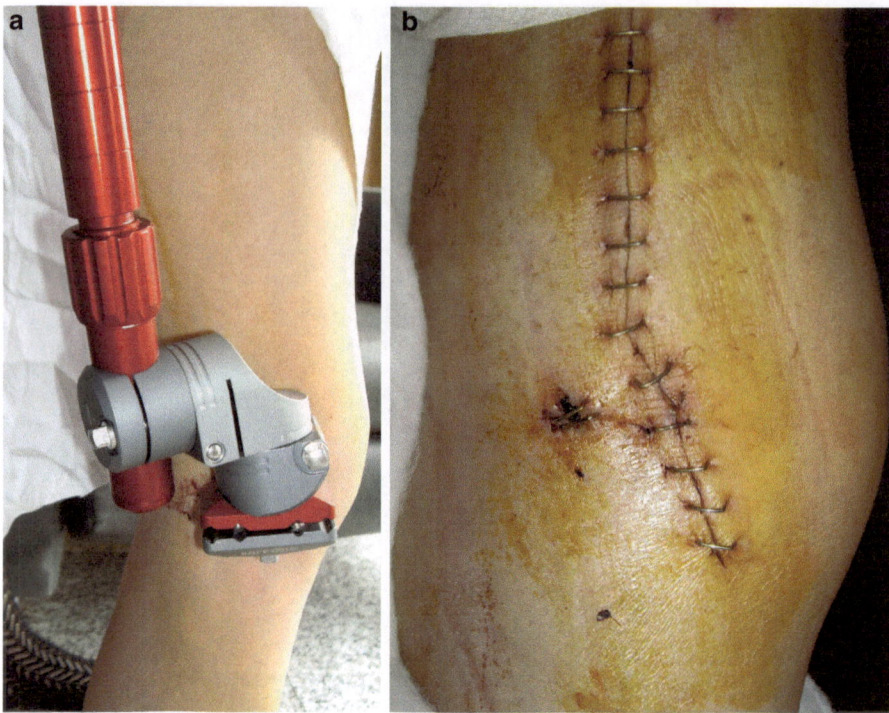

Fig. 9.7 (**a**) The risk of infection is not higher because the external fixator is only in place for 10–15 days. (**b**) In this case, one pin tract was removed in the surgical approach

Incorporation of Graft

Before 1986, as we did not have a bone bank, we used autografts from the ipsilateral or contralateral tibia, and iliac crests (Fig. 9.8). Since that date, we have used allografts[23] in most cases.[30–32]

The use of autografts resulted in an average of 2.8 operations per patient before graft consolidation.[5,39] With allografts, this average was reduced to 0.74. Consolidation at the metaphysis occurred before 6 months had elapsed, but at the diaphyseal end, it often took longer than a year. In metaphyseal unions, we used several types of osteosynthesis devices, such as Kirschner wires, Enders, screws, and staples. Diaphyseal osteotomy and osteosynthesis devices are discussed at the end of this chapter.

Since 1987, at the University Clinic of Navarra, we have used 413 massive bone allografts in the conservative treatment of malignant bone tumours. The allograft type depended on how the cartilage growth plate was affected and on the possibilities of preserving the joint near the tumour.

We did monthly radiological follow-ups during the first year of systemic chemotherapy, with diagnostic studies to assess the local and systemic control of disease. Afterwards, follow-ups were every 3 months for another year, and subsequently every 6 months. In all

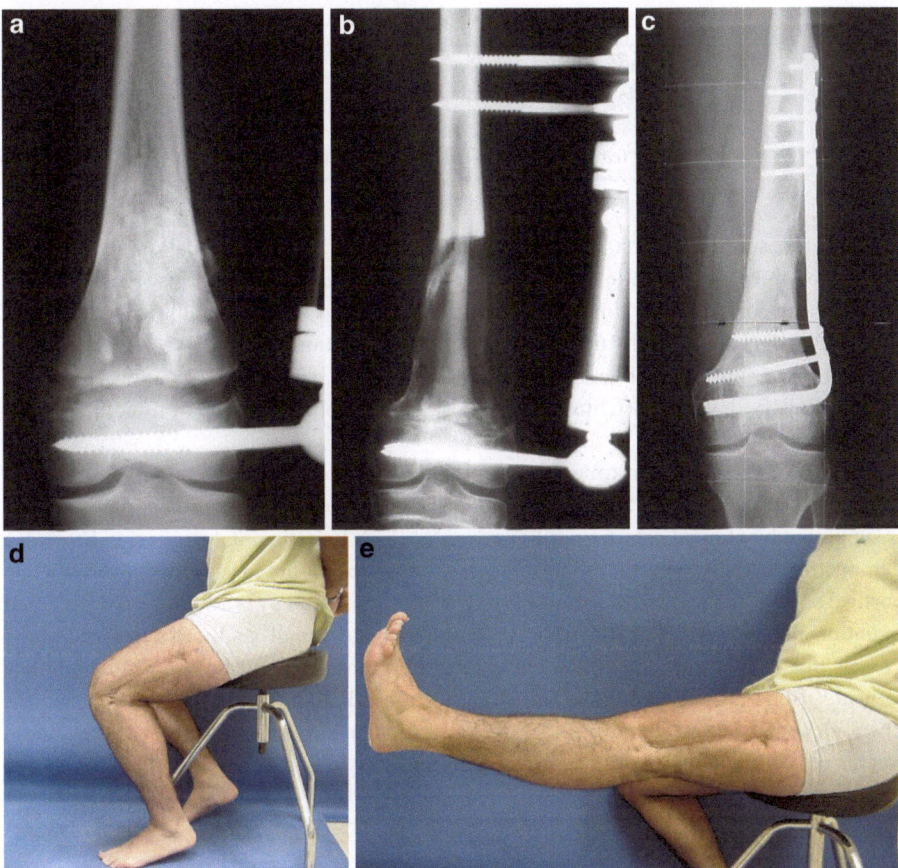

Fig. 9.8 (**a**) Radiograph showing an osteosarcoma of the femur in a 14-year-old boy after physeal distraction. (**b**) After resection of the tumour and autografting from the left tibia. The same frame was used for stabilizing the graft. (**c**) Twenty-two years later, the knee joint has an excellent aspect. (**d, e**) The function of the knee remains excellent. This patient plays sports without restrictions

cases, chemotherapy and radiotherapy were in accordance with the University Clinic of Navarra Cancer Protocol[34,35] for the type of tumour.

Radiological Study

We used the ISOLS criteria (Table 9.1) to evaluate consolidation results,[18] and analysed the following factors which can influence consolidation: host and donor age, allograft length and location, osteotomy and osteosynthesis type, intra-arterial and systemic chemotherapy, and intra-operative and external radiotherapy. We performed a multi-variant statistical analysis, with the Stat-view program.

The mean consolidation time of metaphyseal osteotomies (including those cases in which physeal distraction was used before excision of the tumour) was 6.5 months; none

Table 9.1 ISOLS criteria regarding fusion of allografts

Excellent: Fusion complete. Osteotomy line not visible
Good: Fusion >75%. Osteotomy line still visible
Fair: Fusion 25–75%
Poor: Fusion <25%. No evidence of callus

of the factors studied had a statistically significant influence on consolidation. In metaphyseal osteotomies, consolidation was achieved with minimal osteosynthesis (Fig. 9.9).

The mean consolidation time of diaphyseal osteotomies was 16 months (Fig. 9.10). We found no statistically significant differences in consolidation with the use of intra-arterial chemotherapy, intra-operative radiotherapy, donor age, osteosynthesis type (plates vs intra-medullary devices), osteotomy type (horizontal vs oblique), type of tumour, or location of the tumour.

The mean consolidation time of metaphyseal osteotomies (6.5 months) is similar to that reported by others.[14,38] Systemic chemotherapy delayed consolidation and this finding is supported by clinical data from other series.[8–10,15,36,37] Experimental studies[13,41] have also demonstrated that chemotherapeutic agents impair bone healing, and that allogeneic cortical bone grafts incorporate more slowly when chemotherapy is administered. External radiation also delayed consolidation. Radiation damages small- and medium-sized blood vessels that supply nutrients to the bone, making it more difficult for the irradiated bone to heal.[11] Bone growth retardation resulting from irradiation is clearly a dose-dependent phenomenon.[1,12,20,40] We believe that if the fracture of an allograft can heal with a standard treatment for fractures, it is because the allograft is revascularized at the time of the fracture.[22]

Isotopic Study

A prospective isotopic study was performed[25] in 36 patients with 99mTc MDP in order to evaluate the revascularization of the allografts. Bone scintigraphy with 99mTc HDP was performed 3 h after injection. Anterior and posterior views over both limbs were evaluated qualitatively by two physicians. Semi-quantitative measurements were performed with a region of interest technique. Labelling was scored by area: over bone allograft, A1; over the area just above the allograft, A2; over the opposite limb in the same place as A1 and A2, A3 and A4, respectively. Background over soft tissues was considered and subtracted from all the regions of interest. The allograft uptake was related with the uptake over A2 and A3, and two indices were obtained: $I1 = A1/A2$ and $I2 = A1/A3$. A further index, $A2/A4$, was also calculated.

All patients showed objective uptake of the 99mTc-MDP (Fig. 9.11). The values of the allograft/host bone index were conditioned by the allograft site and by the analysed areas. As in normal bone, uptake at the metaphysis and the epiphysis was greater than in the diaphysis. Areas over an allograft with an intra-medullary nail showed less uptake than the contralateral area. In areas near an allograft, uptake was greater surrounding the osteosynthesis device, due to increased metabolism. In most cases, the allograft-host bone junction

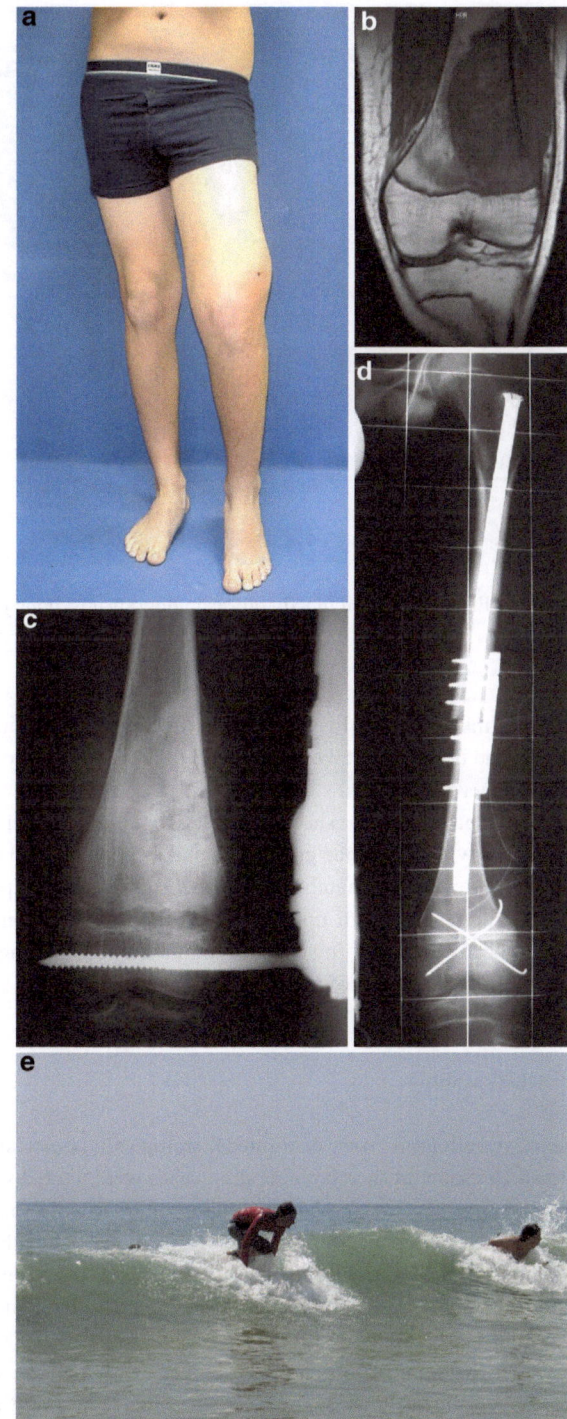

Fig. 9.9 (**a**, **b**) Osteosarcoma in the distal metaphysis of the femur of a 14-year-old boy. (**c**) Physeal distraction was performed and (**d**) an intercalary allograft was used for reconstruction. The healing at the distal junction was achieved with two Kirschner wires, while the diaphyseal junction required stronger osteosynthesis. (**e**) The same patient surfing

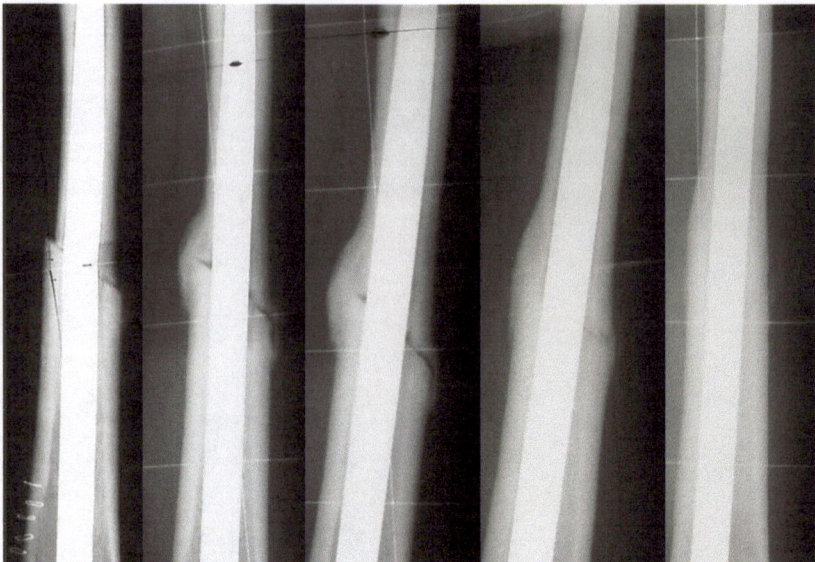

Fig. 9.10 Excellent fusion in a diaphyseal allograft-host bone junction

showed more uptake. Five patients suffered a fracture in their allografts, but no relation was found between uptake indices and the risk of fracture. Uptake was greater in allografts with longer follow-ups.

The isotopic study showed objective uptake in all the allografts, and this uptake increased with time since grafting. Uptake can be related to allograft revascularization and demonstrates active metabolism in the allograft. The uptake pattern is similar to that of normal bone. The high uptake at the allograft-host bone junction in cases subjected to study shortly after grafting can be explained by the healing process. This study also allowed us to evaluate activity of the retained growth plate (Fig. 9.11).

Histological Study

Retrieved allografts were examined histologically, especially at the allograft-host bone junction area. Some of the corresponding cases were treated with tetracyclines (Tetra-Hubber®) for 4–6 days before removal of the allograft in order to study the allograft incorporation.

In all cases, the healing process at the allograft-host bone junction involved periosteal callus from the receptor bone (Fig. 9.12). Histological examination of allografts revealed necrotic bone, except in the areas near the host bone, and an external surface invaded by vascular buds from adjacent soft tissue.

Apart from showing healing progressing by periosteal callus, the histological studies confirmed the features of the isotopic study regarding the revascularization of allografts from the surrounding tissue.

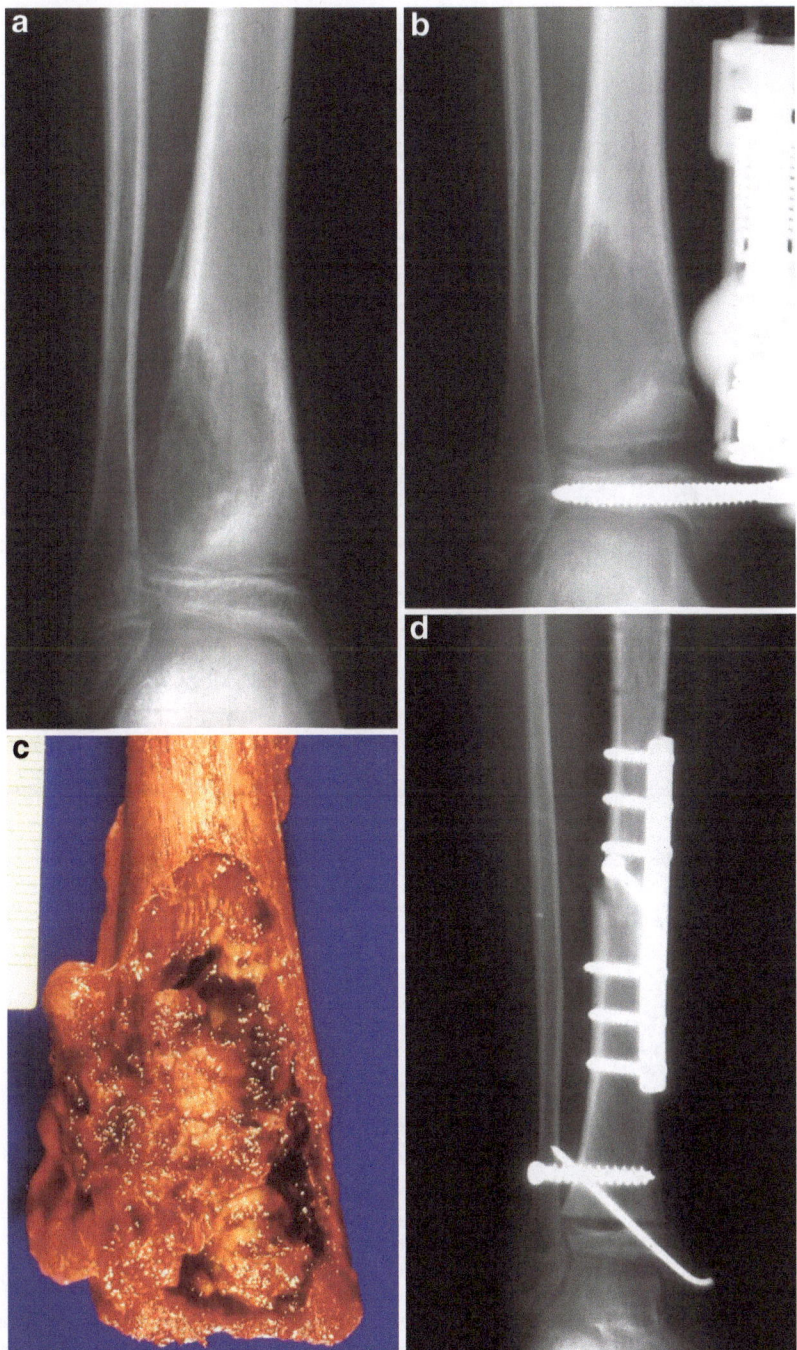

Fig. 9.11 (**a**) Telangiectatic osteosarcoma in the distal tibia of a 10-year-old girl. (**b**) Physeal distraction was performed before excision (**c**) of the tumour. (**d**) Reconstruction was carried out with an intercalary allograft.

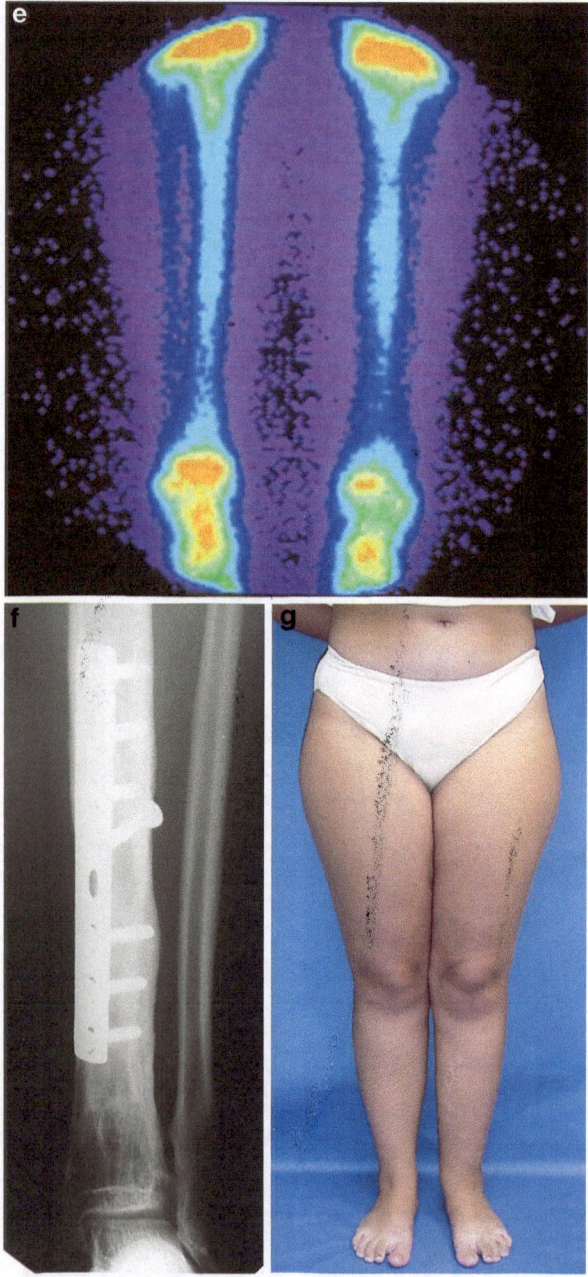

Fig. 9.11 (continued) (**e**) Three years after surgery, the growth plate remains active. Isotopic uptake in the allograft is similar to that in the contralateral tibia. (**f, g**) This patient has no dissymmetry 12 years after treatment

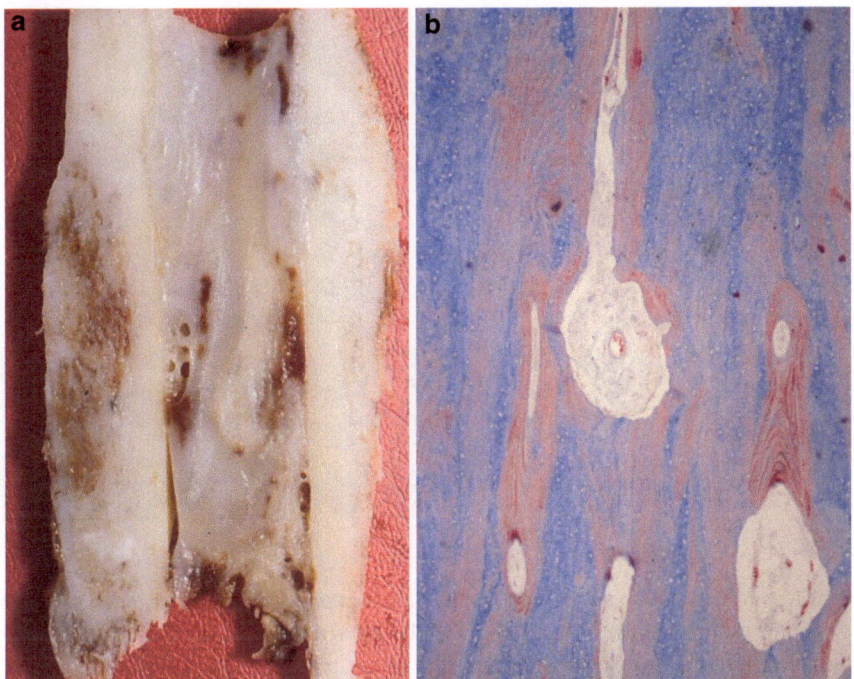

Fig. 9.12 (**a**) Macroscopic image of the periosteal callus at the allograft-host bone junction. (**b**) Masson's trichrome staining of a retrieved allograft, showing vessels into the cortex of the graft

Subsequent Growth

When treating a bone sarcoma, an orthopaedic surgeon's first concern is to preserve the life of the patient. In most cases, the surgeon can also preserve the limb, although there is little sense in preserving a limb if will be non-functional. Better functional results are achieved when the joint of the patient can be preserved. When considering how to conserve functionality, it also necessary to bear in mind the future growth of the limb.

Subsequent growth of a limb is not only affected by the surgical technique employed in terms of the resection of one or more growth plates. Even in cases where the growth plate is left intact, the osteosynthesis device or radiotherapy[16–18,33] could cause arrest of growth (Fig. 9.13). In addition, high doses of chemotherapy have been reported as a cause of decrease in GH secretion.

In the last few years, various different methods to preserve the joint of a patient with a metaphyseal bone tumour have been described. Physeal distraction before excision of the tumour, as described by Cañadell in 1984, has, in our opinion, the advantage of safety: the growth plate is not a flat plane, but an irregular surface, and therefore an intra-epiphyseal osteotomy could leave parts of the tumour. Furthermore, with Cañadell's physeal distraction, the whole epiphysis can be preserved, thereby increasing the joint's stability; facilitating resection and osteosynthesis of the graft; and avoiding damage to the femoropatellar joint

Fig. 9.13 This Ewing's sarcoma in the proximal left tibia was treated by pre-operative radiotherapy. Note the limits of the irradiation field in comparison with the right tibia. The preservation of this growth plate would not prevent a limb-length discrepancy

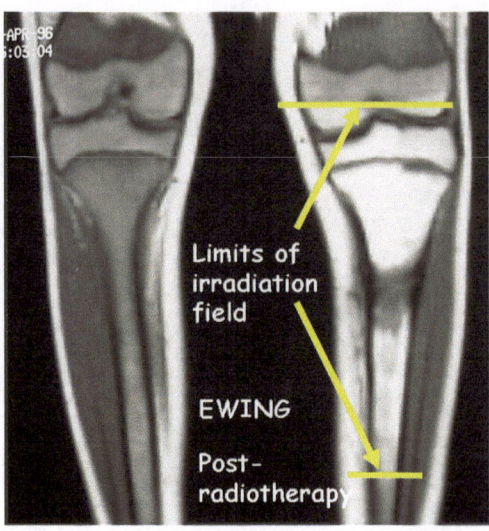

in distal femur tumours, patellar tendon attachment in proximal tibia tumours, or the rotator cuff in proximal humerus tumours. Finally, physeal distraction before excision can preserve most of the growth plate because the physis breaks in the metaphyseal border of the growth plate as a result of the degenerative lack of cells there (Figs. 9.14–9.16).

Physeal distraction is indicated in cases of metaphyseal bone tumours in children when the growth plate is still open and the surgeon is sure that the tumour has not invaded the epiphysis. Other applications for external fixation in tumoural cases include distraction callostasis for limb-length discrepancy, tumour resection and bone transport, combined distraction callostasis and compression for limb-length discrepancy, and concurrent diaphyseal non-union.

Distraction callostasis[21] was indicated in patients with serious dissymmetry (more than 4 cm) who had been free of disease for at least 3 years after the first limb salvage procedure.[6] The average age for this procedure was $10 + 7$ years. Other patients with limb-length discrepancy had equalization by other means, such as epiphysiodesis on the contralateral limb or changing of the allograft (Fig. 9.17). The mean length gained was 9.5 cm (in the range of 7–12 cm) with an average healing index of 34 days/cm. The Mankin limb function grade was excellent or good in 63% of the cases.

When the growth plate cannot be preserved, it is more difficult to avoid dissymmetry (Fig. 9.18).

Osteosynthesis of Grafts in Children

Osteosynthesis of the allograft should be borne in mind in order to prevent a final limb-length discrepancy.

Previous studies in our department[24] showed that whatever the osteosynthesis device used, consolidation in the metaphysis occurred before 6 months. At the diaphyseal end,

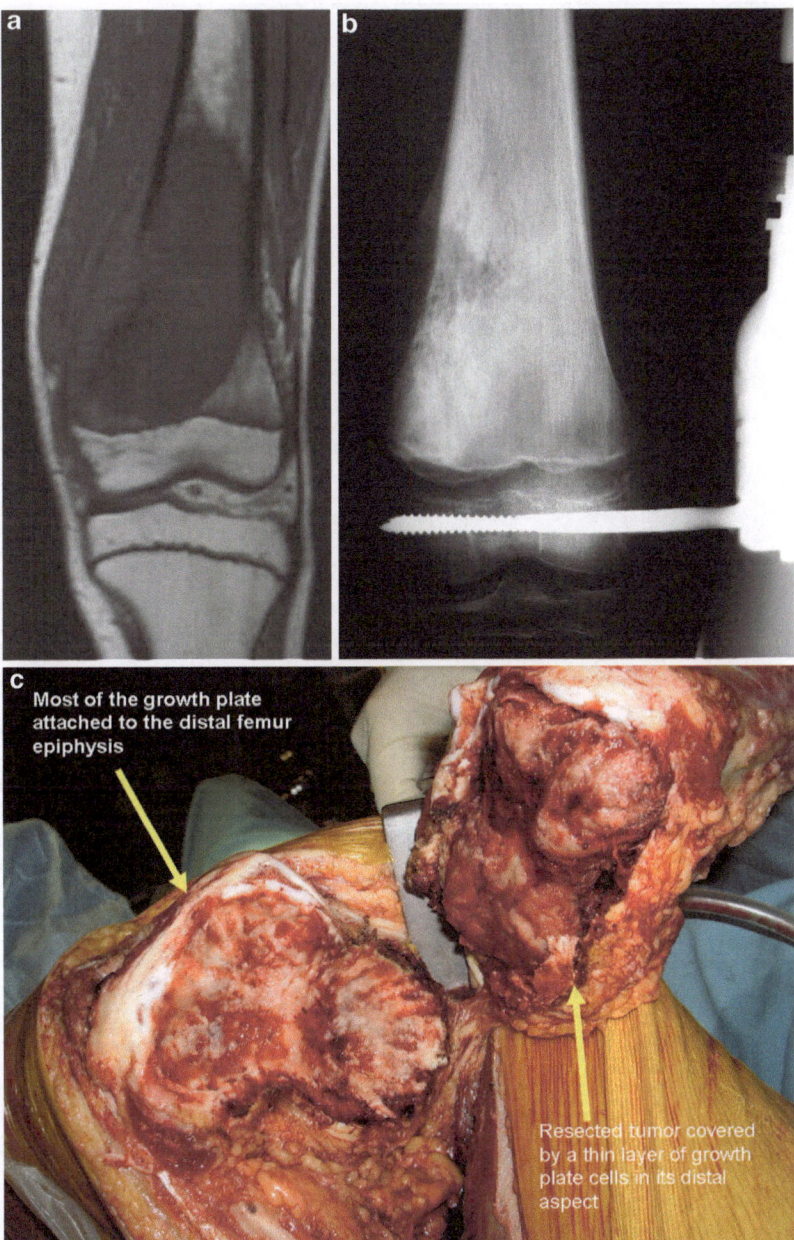

Fig. 9.14 (**a**) This osteosarcoma in the distal femur does not involve the growth plate, as shown on the MRI. (**b**) Epiphysiolysis was performed. (**c**) Intra-operative view during resection showing the epiphysis covered by a white surface, the growth plate, preservation of which can allow potential for growth. A thin layer of growth plate cells covers the resected tumour, and this constitutes a wide margin. Note the undulations in the growth plate

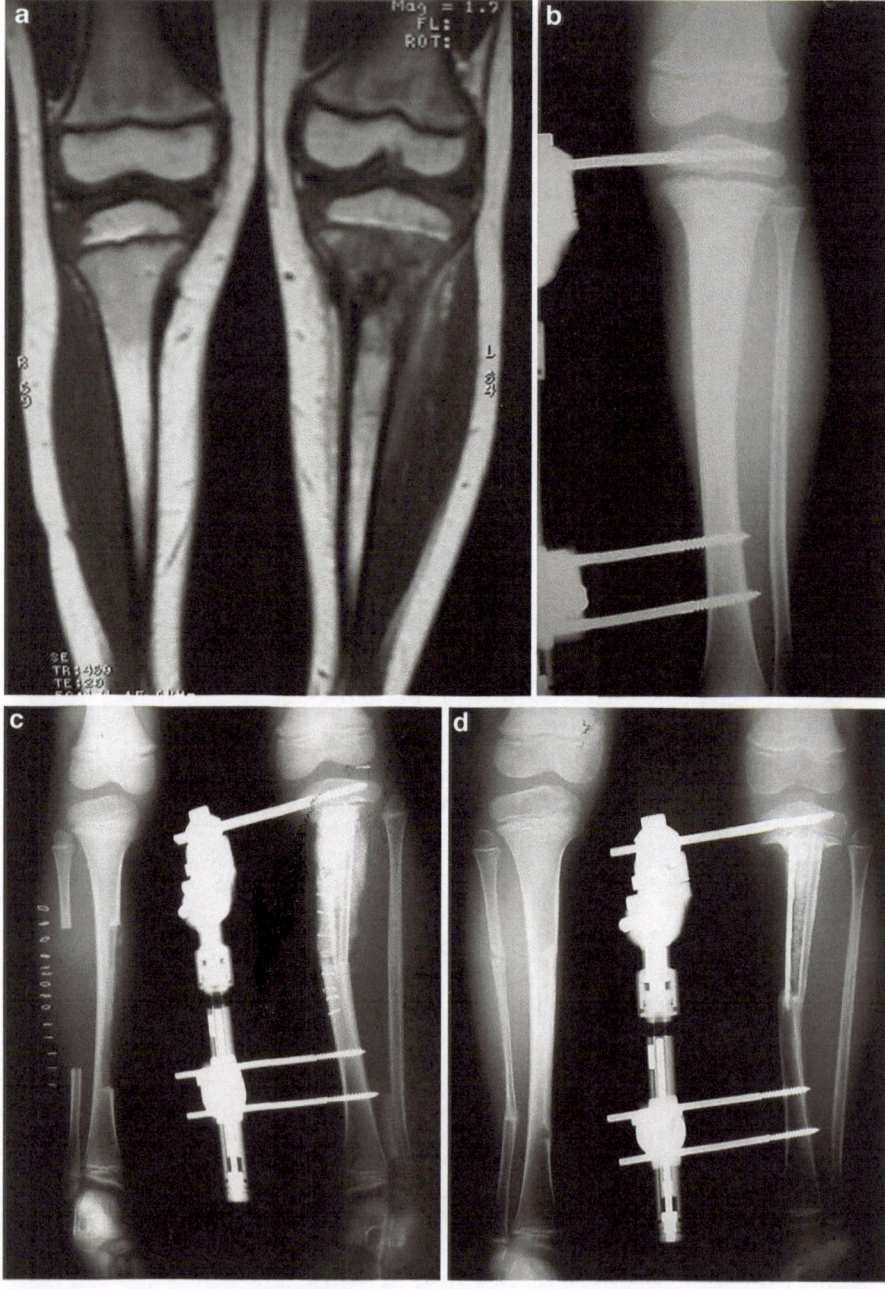

Fig. 9.15 (**a**) A Ewing's sarcoma in the proximal metaphysis of the left tibia of a 4-year-old girl. (**b**) After distraction (**c**), reconstruction was performed with an autograft from the contralateral tibia and fibula. (**d**) After healing of the graft, the external fixator was removed. Details of the preserved growth plate after resection

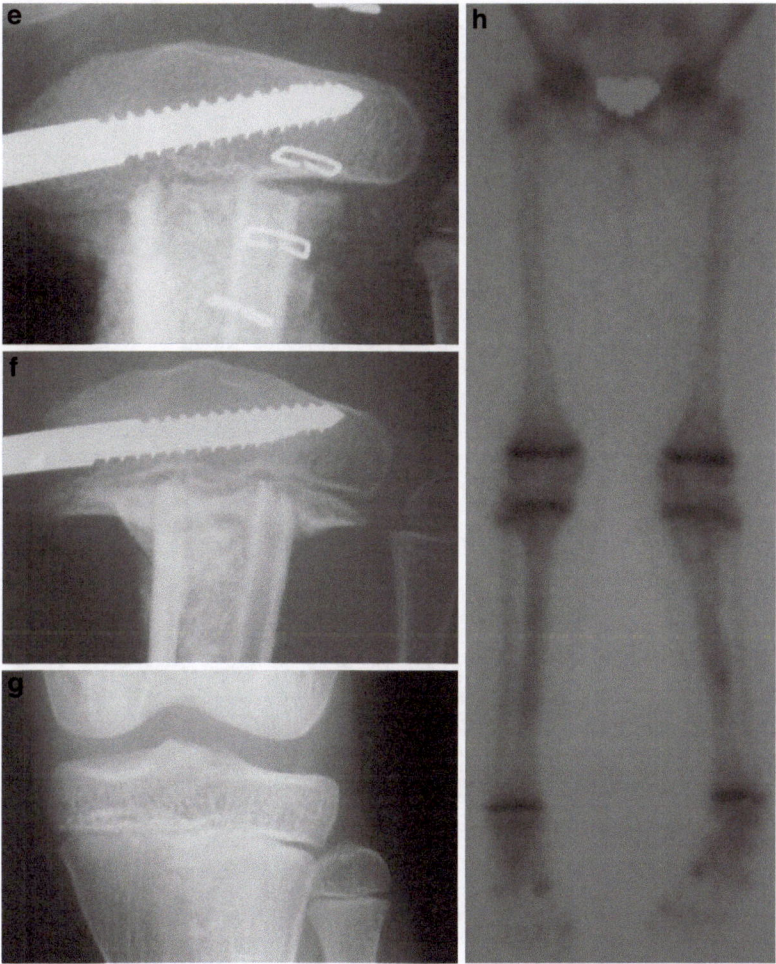

Fig. 9.15 (continued) (**e**), after healing of the graft (**f**), and 4 years later (**g**), showing normal growth. (**h**) Bone scan showing normal uptake in the distracted physis, 4 years post-operative therapy

however, consolidation often took over a year. In addition, the "osteosynthesis *ad minimum* law" is not applicable, even in children, at the diaphyseal union when allografts are used. On the other hand, fractures of allografts are more often seen when non-intra-medullary devices are used for stabilization at the allograft-host bone union.[22] Therefore, we prefer the use of locked, intra-medullary nails for stabilization of allografts; the nail should be locked in the epiphysis in cases of preservation of the joint. However, the locked nail will not allow growth from the preserved growth plate.

Minimal osteosynthesis devices, for example, Kirschner wires, are enough to stabilize the metaphyseal junction, and present no problems in terms of achieving union, but will not allow early mobilization of the joint.

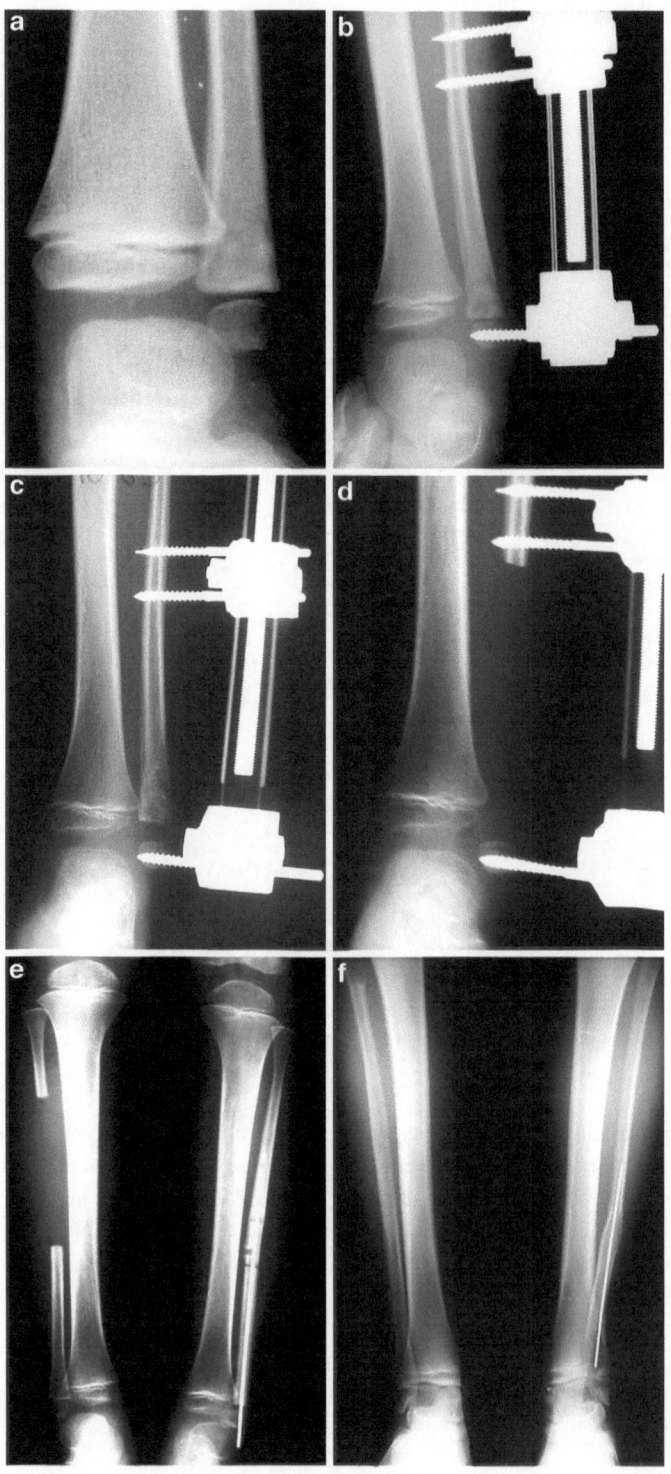

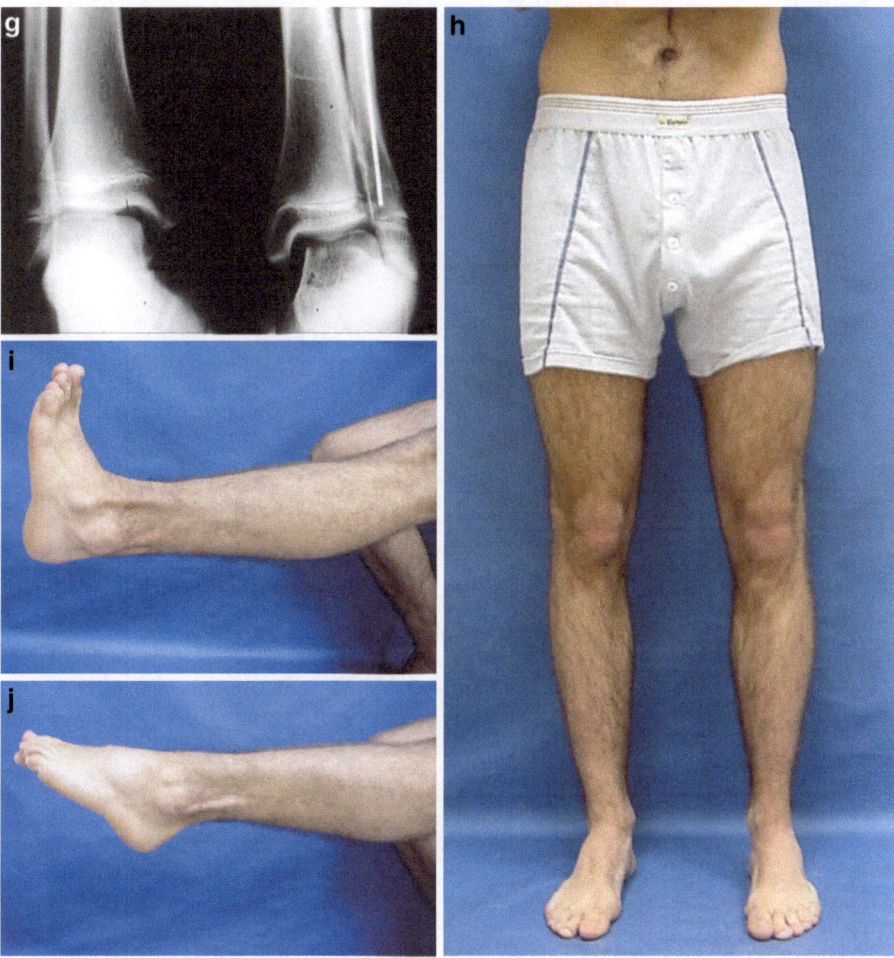

Fig. 9.16 (a) A Ewing's sarcoma in the distal metaphysis of the left fibula of a 4-year-old boy. In 1985, given the age of the patient, many orthopaedic surgeons would have considered an amputation. (b, c) However, we performed a physeal distraction. (d) The tumour was resected, and the external fixator was maintained until histological assessment corroborated that the tumour did not involve the growth plate: in 1985, MRI was not available. (e) The limb was reconstructed with a graft. Note the Kirschner wire protruding a few centimetres below the joint. (f) Twelve years later, the ankle was still normal. The Kirschner wire has gone up, demonstrating the normal growth of this physis. (g) This is a comparative X-ray of the two ankles taken in 2007. (h–j) After 22 years, the patient has no dissymmetry and function is normal; the patient plays soccer for his local village team

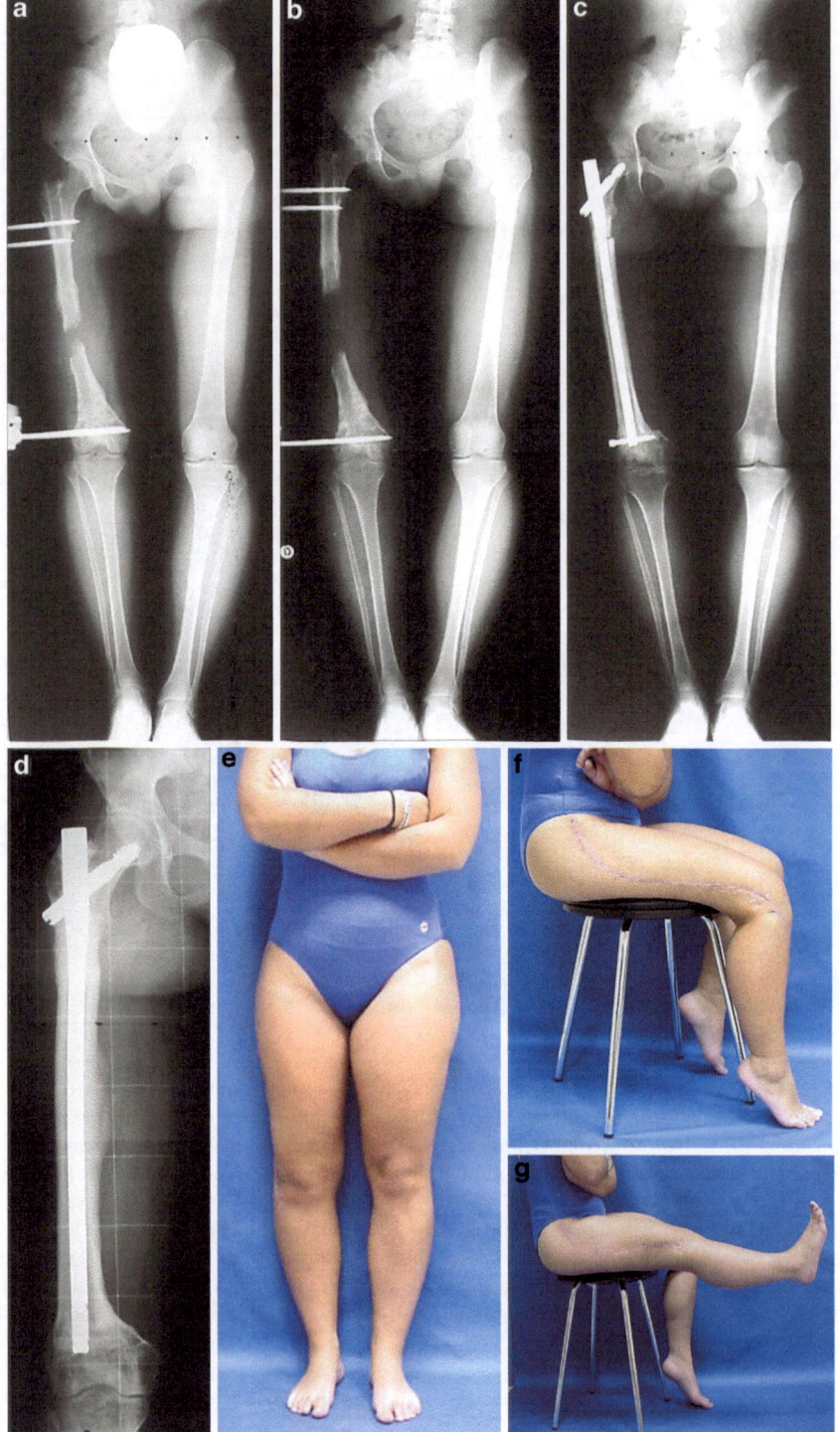

Fig. 9.17 Limb-length discrepancy 6 years after intercalary reconstruction of an osteosarcoma in the distal metaphysis of the femur of an 8-year-old girl. (**a**) The osteosynthesis device was removed and distraction was performed through the shaft of the allograft. After discrepancy was corrected (**b**), a new allograft was implanted (**c**). The allograft healed (**d**) and function was excellent (**e-g**)

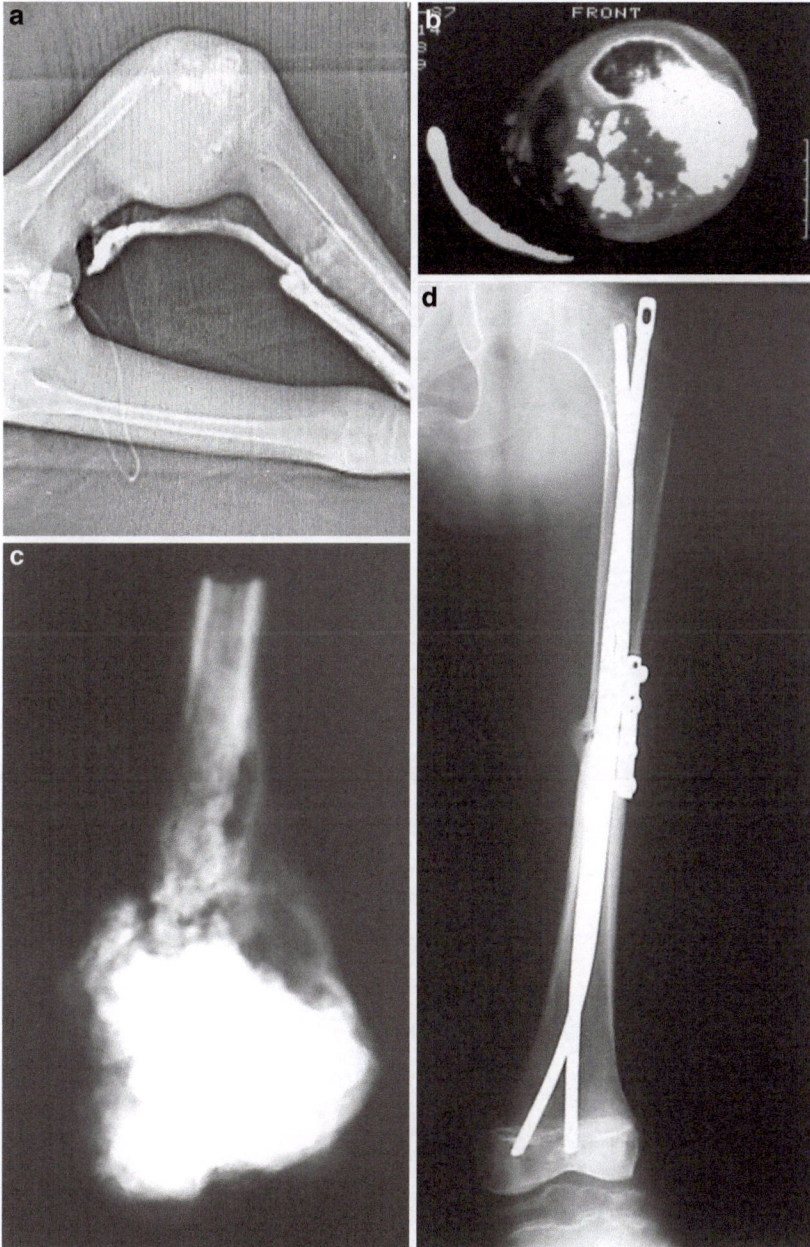

Fig. 9.18 (a, b) An 8-year-old boy with a large osteosarcoma on his left femur. (c) The tumour was resected, (d) and the limb was reconstructed with an osteoarticular allograft.

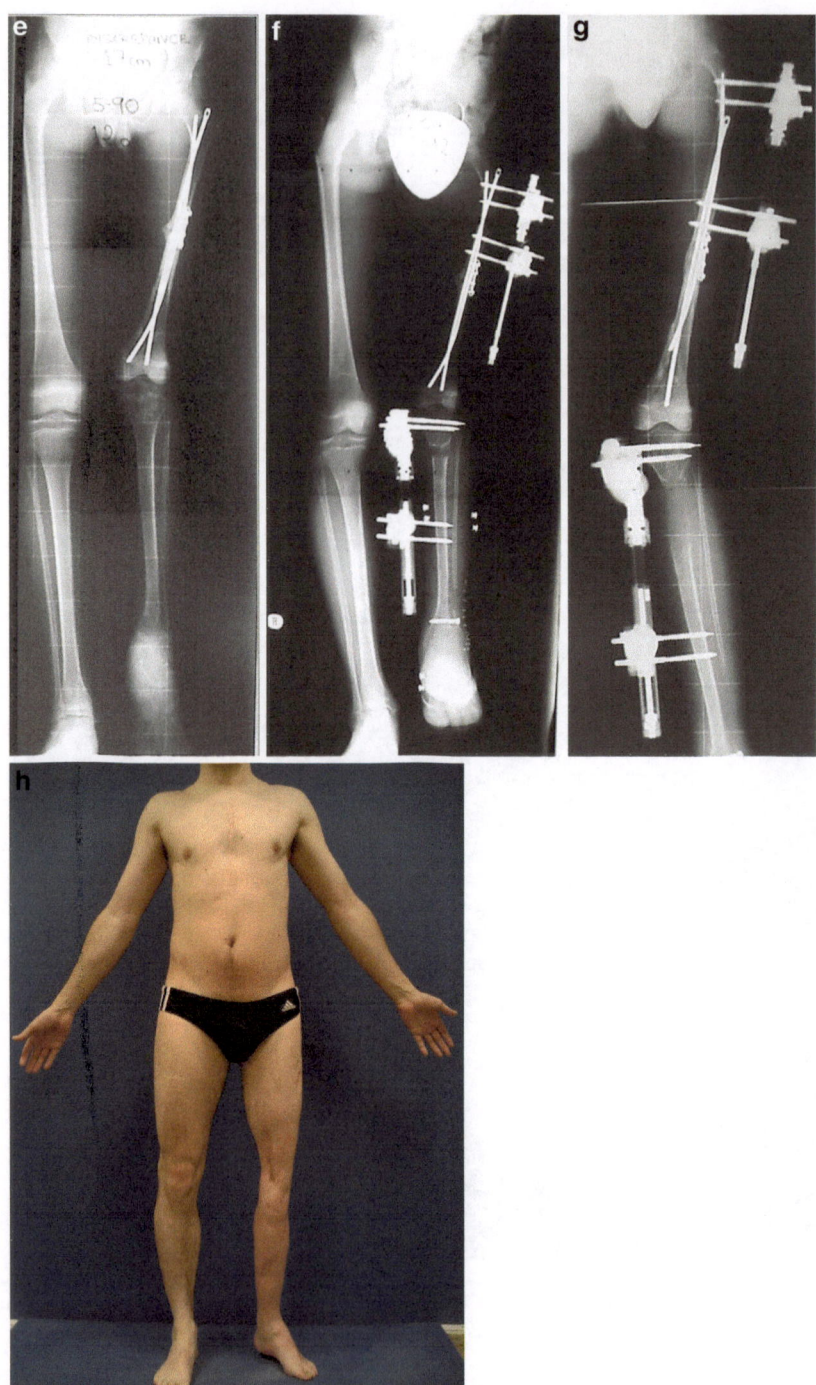

Fig. 9.18 (continued) (**e**) Over time, a leg-length discrepancy developed. (**f, g**) After 5 years, we performed bone lengthening in both the femur and the tibia. (**h**) The patient is alive and free of disease 21 years after the first limb salvage procedure

In summary, the osteosynthesis device at the diaphyseal union should be stable enough to achieve union, and, in order to avoid fracture of the allograft, intra-medullary nails are preferable. Healing at the metaphyseal union can be achieved with much simpler osteosynthesis devices, which could preserve the potential for growth but will not allow for early mobilization of the joint. Therefore, when the patient is near the end of growth or radiotherapy has been or will be used, we recommend the use of locked intra-medullary nails (with a locking screw in the retained epiphysis) and an allograft longer than the resected piece. In young patients, a very simple osteosynthesis device could be used at the metaphyseal junction in order to preserve the growth potential of the retained growth plate.

Conclusion

In young children, physeal distraction prior to limb salvage is a viable and safe way to preserve normal joint. In our series of such patients with a metaphyseal tumour and intact physis, subsequent limb function was graded as excellent or good in two-thirds of cases. The use of this technique does not increase the rate of local or distant tumour spread. The majority of complications encountered are due to difficulties inherent in reconstruction with structural bone grafts. We have also successfully used distraction callatosis for leg-length discrepancy following limb salvage. In our series of patients, complications and healing rates after distraction callatasis are similar to those with standard lengthening procedures. In selected cases of leg-length discrepancy and non-union, external fixation may be used to compress and heal the non-union site while lengthening at another.

References

1. Bisgardt JD, Hunt HB. Influence of roentgen rays and radium on epiphyseal growth of long bones. *Radiology*, 1936;26:56.
2. Cañadell J, San Julian M. Tumoral reconstruction in the immature knee. In: De Pablos, ed. The Immature Knee. Masson, Barcelona; 1998:343–349.
3. Cañadell J, San Julian M, Forriol F, Cara JA. Physeal distraction in the conservative treatment of malignant bone tumors in children. In: De Pablos, ed. Surgery of the Growth Plate. Madrid: Ergon; 1998:321–327.
4. Cañadell J, San Julian M. Cirugía de salvamento en el tratamiento de los tumores óseos malignos En: Guillen P, ed. *Evolución de la Traumatología y la Ortopedia en los últimos 25 años: ¡Un cuarto de siglo!*. Fundación Mapfre Medicina; 1999: 687–692.
5. Cara JA, Amillo S, Cañadell J. Bone grafts in the treatment of malignant bone tumors: autografts vs. allografts. In: Cañadell J, San-Julian M, Cara JA, eds. *Surgical Treatment of Malignant Bone Tumors*. Orthopaedic monographies. Pamplona: Universidad de Navarra; 1995:111–120.
6. Cara JA, Cañadell J, Forriol F. Bone lengthening after conservative oncologic surgery. In: Cañadell J, San-Julian M, Cara JA, eds. *Surgical Treatment of Malignant Bone Tumors*. Orthopaedic monographies. Pamplona: Universidad de Navarra; 1995:215–225.
7. Cara JA, San-Julian M, Laclériga A, and Cañadell J. Infection in grafting procedures. In: Cañadell J, San-Julian M, Cara JA, eds. *Surgical Treatment of Malignant Bone Tumors*. Orthopaedic monographies. Pamplona: Universidad de Navarra; 1995:227–234.

8. Delépine N, Delépine G, Hernigou PH, Desbois J. Bone union of allografts and chemotherapy considerations about 55 consecutive cases. *Fifth International Symposium on Limb Salvage*. St Malo, 5, 1989.
9. Dyck H, Malinin T, Mnaymneh W. Massive allograft implantation following radical resection of high grade tumors requiring neoadjuvant chemotherapy treatment. *Clin Orthop*. 1988;197:88.
10. Glasser DB, Duane K, Lane JM, Healey JH, Caparros-Sison B. The effect of chemotherapy on growth in the skeletally immature individual. *Clin Orthop*. 1991;262:93–107.
11. Goldwein JW. Effects of radiation therapy in skeletal growth in childhood. *Clin Orthop*. 1991;262:101–107.
12. Gonzales DG, Van Dijk, JD. Experimental studies on the response of growing bones to X-ray and neutron irradiation. *Int J Radiot Oncol Biol Phys*. 1991;9:671.
13. Khoo DB. The effect of chemotherapy on soft tissue and bone healing in the rabbit model. *Ann Acad Med Singapore*. 1992;21:217–221.
14. Mankin H, Springfield D, Gebhart M, Tomford W. Current status of allografting for bone tumors. *Orthopedics*. 1992;15:1147–1154.
15. Mnaymneh W, Malinin T, Lackman R, Hornicek J, Ghandur-Mnaimneh L. Massive distal femoral allografts after resection of bone tumors. *Clin Orthop*. 1994;303:103–115.
16. Martinez-Monge R, Cambeiro M, San-Julian M, Sierrasesúmaga L. The use of braquitherapy in paediatric cancer: the search of an uncomplicated cure. *Lancet Oncol*. February 2006;7(2):157–166.
17. Martinez-Monge R, San Julian M, Amillo S, et al. Perioperative high dose brachytherapy in high-risk resected sarcomas: initial results of a Phase I/II Trial. *Radiotherapy*. 2004.
18. Martinez Monge R, Garrán C, Cambeiro M, San-Julian M, Alcalde J, Sierrasesúmaga L. Feasibility Report of Conservative Surgery, Perioperative HDR brachytherapy (PHDRB) and low to moderate esternal beam radiation therapy (EBRT) in pediatric sarcomas. *Brachytherapy* 2004;3:196–200.
19. Neel M, Bush C, Scarborough M, Enneking W. Transepiphyseal extension of osteosarcoma. Abstract book of the 8th ISOLS (International Symposium on Limb Salvage), Florence, May 10th-12th, 1995;107.
20. Rosen G, Caparros B, Niremberg A, et al. Ewing's sarcoma. Ten years experience with adyuvant chemotherapy. *Cancer*, 1981;47:2204–2213.
21. San-Julián M, Cañadell J. Physeal distraction and bone lengthening in young children with malignant bone tumors. *Acta Orthop Sand*. 1997;Suppl 276:68.
22. San-Julian M, Cañadell J. Fractures in allografts for limb preserving operations. *Int Orthop*. 1998;22:32–36.
23. San-Julián M, Amillo S, Cañadell J. Allografts in malignant bone tumors. In: Czitrom AA, Winkler H, eds. Orthopaedic allograft surgery. New York: Springer Wien; 1996: 157–163.
24. San-Julián M, Leyes M, Mora G, Cañadell J. Consolidation of massive bone allografts in limb preserving operations for bone tumors. *Int Orthop*. 1995;19:377–382.
25. San-Julián M, Villas A, Cañadell J, Ricther JA. Allograft revascularization scintigraphic study with 99m Tc MDP. Abstract book of the IX meeting of European Musculo Skeletal Oncology Society. Instambul, Turkiye; 24–25 October 1996:14.
26. San Julian M, Diaz de Rada P, Noain E, Sierrasesúmaga L. Bone metastases from osteosarcoma. *Int Orthop*. 2003;27(2):117–120.
27. San Julian M. Tumores óseos malignos en la edad infantil. En: De Pablos J, Bruguera A, eds. Apuntes de Ortopedia infantil, 2nd edición. Pamplona: Ergón; 2000.
28. San Julian M, Cara JA, Cañadell J. Is amputation still really neccesary in any case of osteosarcoma? *Rev Med Univ Navarra*. 1999;43:13–25.
29. San Julian M, Dolz R, Garcia-Barrecheguren E, Noain E, Sierrasesumaga L, J Cañadell. Limb salvage in bone sarcomas in patients younger than age 10: A 20 years experience." *Am J Pediat Orthopaed*. Nov-Dec 2003;6(23):753–762.

30. San Julian M, Forriol F, Cañadell J. Investigación en banco de tejidos osteoarticulares Monografias SECOT 4: Banco de huesos. Masson; 2002:69–79.
31. San Julian M, Valentí A. Bone transplant. Transplante de órganos y tejidos. *Anales del Sistema navarro de Salud*. 2006;28(Suppl 2):125–136.
32. San Julian M, Moreno JL, Forriol F, Cañadell J. Integración radiológica, isotópica e histológica de los aloinjertos corticales. Estudio clínico. *Rev Ortop Traum*. 2000;44:436–441.
33. San Julian M, Aristu J. Sarcoma de Ewing. Luis Sierrasesúmaga. En: Antillon F, Patiño A, Bernaola E, San Julian M, eds. *Oncología Pediátrica. Luis Sierrasesúmaga*. Madrid: Pearson; 2005:617–636.
34. Sierrasesúmaga L, Antillón F, Cañadell J. Treatment of Ewing's sarcoma. Protocol, description, applications and results. In: Cañadell J, Sierrasesúmaga L, Calvo F, Ganoza C, eds. *Treatment of Malignant Bone Tumors in Children and adolescents*. Pamplona: Servicio de Publicaciones de la Universidad de Navarra S.A; 1991.
35. Sierrasesúmaga L, Antillón F, Cañadell J. Treatment of Osteosarcoma. Protocol, description, applications and results. In: Cañadell J, Sierrasesúmaga L, Calvo F, Ganoza C, eds. *Treatment of Malignant Bone Tumors in Children and Adolescents*. Pamplona: Servicio de Publicaciones de la Universidad de Navarra S.A.; 1991.
36. Silverman EN. The skeletal lesions in leukemia: clinical and roentgenographic observations in 103 infants and children, with a review of the literature. *AJR*. 1948;59:818.
37. Sinohara N, Sumida S, Masuda S. Bone allografts after segmental resection of tumors. *Int Orthop*. 1990;14:273–276.
38. Vander Griend R. The effect of internal fixation on the healing of large allografts. *J Bone Joint Surg*. 1994;76 A:657 664.
39. Villas C, San Julian M, Alfonso M. Autoinjertos en cirugía de los tumores óseos. Injertos, Sustitutivos óseos y materiales en la cirugía reconstructiva del aparato locomotor. Masson; 2005.
40. Whitehouse WM, Lampe I. Osseous damage in irradiation of renal tumors in infancy and childhood. *AJR*. 1953;70:721.
41. Zart DJ, Miya L, Wolff DA, Mackley JT, Stevenson S. The effects of cisplatin on the incorporation of fresh singenic and frozen allogenic cortical bone grafts. *J Orthop Res*. 1993; 11:240–249.

Other Techniques for Epiphyseal Preservation

10

Mikel San-Julian

Abstract In selected cases, the epiphysis could be preserved by intra-epiphyseal osteotomy, and although physeal distraction before excision of the tumour has some advantages, in some cases osteotomy is indicated.

Introduction

Prior to the first publications of our work, the possibility of preservation of the epiphysis in metaphyscal bone tumours would seem to have been a possibility which was largely overlooked, and alternative techniques, such as intra-epiphyseal osteotomy,[1] have only been suggested subsequently. We have used intra-epiphyseal osteotomy in some cases, in which epiphysis could be preserved but physeal distraction was contraindicated (Figs. 10.1 and 10.2).

In the more recent reports of intra-epiphyseal osteotomy, the technique has been used mainly in proximal tibia locations. Tumour involvement of the physis is assessed by pre-operative MRI. If intra-epiphyseal osteotomy is indicated, it is done under X-ray control in order to include the growth plate in the resected specimen. The residual epiphyseal bone segment is less than 2-cm thick and reconstruction is by a combination of vascularised fibula and allograft.[2] The epiphyseal osteotomy is fixed by small fragment screws.

In our opinion, the advantages of physeal distraction over intra-epiphyseal osteotomy are

1. *Safety*. The growth plate is not a plane surface (Figs. 10.3 and 10.4), but has indentations and protuberances, and consequently an intra-epiphyseal osteotomy could leave bits of tumour.
2. *Easier resection*. Physeal distraction before excision of a metaphyseal bone tumour removes the need for metaphyseal osteotomy. Therefore, resection requires only one osteotomy – the diaphyseal one.
3. *Preservation of the whole epiphysis*. This has several advantages:

Mikel San-Julian
Department of Orthopedic Surgery, University Clinic of Navarra, Avda. Pio XII, s/n, 31008, Pamplona, Navarra, Spain
e-mail: msjulian@unav.es

J. Cañadell and M. San-Julian (eds.), *Pediatric Bone Sarcomas: Epiphysiolysis Before Excision*, DOI: 10.1007/978-1-84882-130-9_10, © Springer-Verlag London Limited 2011

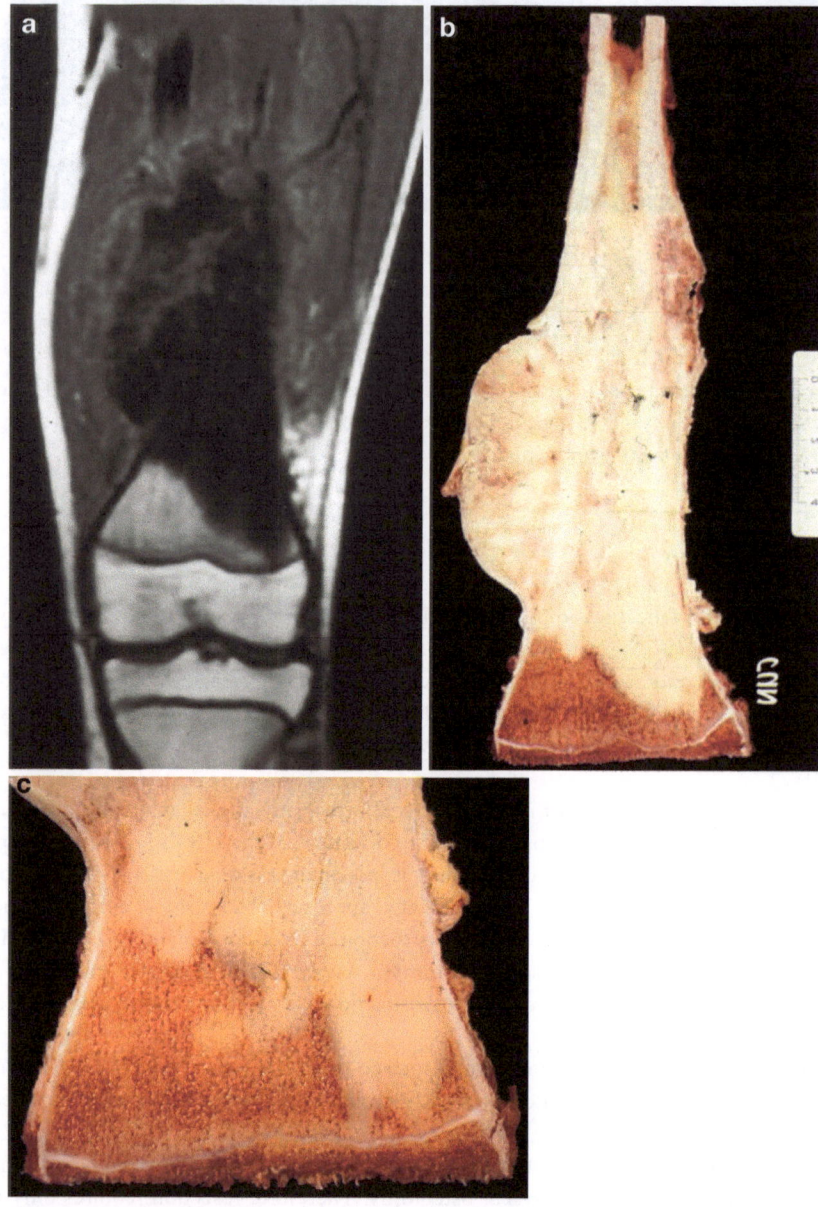

Fig. 10.1 (**a**) Osteosarcoma in the distal metaphysis of the femur of a 16-year-old boy. MRI shows the tumour in contact with the physis. This patient was treated in 1987. (**b**, **c**) Intra-epiphyseal osteotomy was performed in order to preserve the joint. Note that the growth plate is very thin

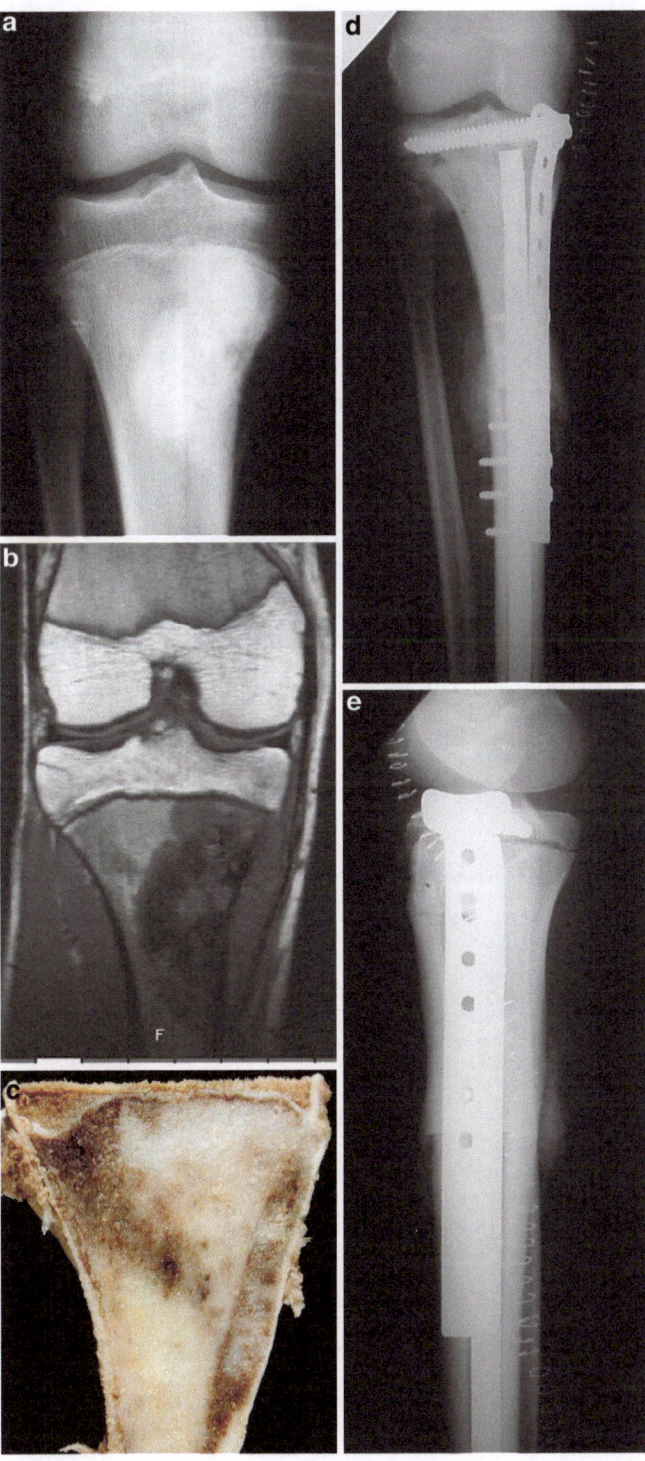

Fig. 10.2 (**a, b**) Osteosarcoma in the proximal metaphysis of the tibia of a 17-year-old boy. The tumour is in contact with the growth plate. (**c**) After careful consideration of epiphysiolysis before resection, we chose intra-epiphyseal osteotomy due to the age of the patient. (**d, e**) Reconstruction with an intercalary allograft stabilised with both a plate and a nail

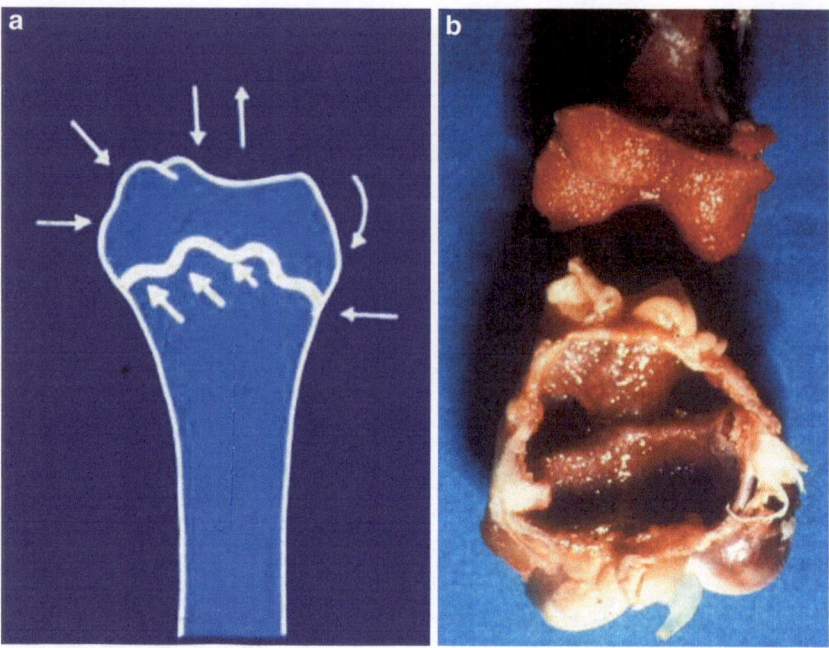

Fig. 10.3 (a) Because of the morphology of the growth plate, intra-epiphyseal osteotomy could leave tumour cells in the hollows of the surface. (b) Experimental epiphysiolysis in a lamb. Note the undulate appearance of the growth plate

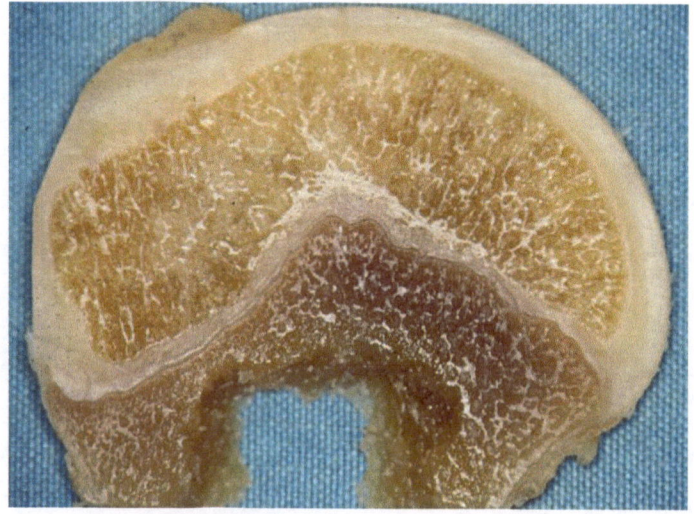

Fig. 10.4 The morphology of the growth plate in the proximal humerus contraindicates, in our opinion, intra-epiphyseal osteotomy

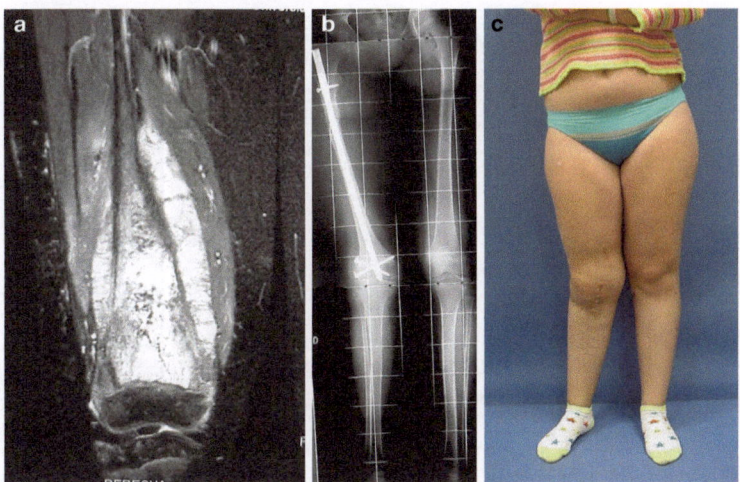

Fig. 10.5 (**a**) Osteosarcoma in contact with the whole physis. (**b**) Intra-epiphyseal osteotomy and reconstruction with an allograft. (**c**) Note the limb length discrepancy and the valgus instability

- Joint stability is better maintained because most ligaments, tendinous attachments, capsules, etc. are preserved (Fig. 10.5).
- Graft osteosynthesis is easier because the epiphyseal segment of bone is bigger.
- In distal femur locations, the *trochlea femoralis* is preserved. Intra-epiphyseal osteotomy implies the loss of part of the *trochlea femoralis* (Fig. 10.6), which can lead to a loss in knee function.

Similarly, the patellar tendon attachment in the proximal tibia (Fig. 10.7) and the rotator cuff in the shoulder can be preserved.

4. ***Preservation of most of the growth plate***. Epiphysiolysis occurs through the layer of degenerative cells on the metaphyseal side of the growth plate. Therefore, most of the growth plate is retained, together with the epiphysis (Fig. 10.8). When the distraction procedure is performed at a rate of 1–1.5 mm/day, the retained physis remains active.[3]

We believe that intra-epiphyseal osteotomy is indicated in the following situations:

- Metaphyseal tumours with no involvement of the physis in which a pathological fracture has occurred. In such cases, physeal distraction is contraindicated because of the risk of distraction through the tumour instead of the growth plate unless the fracture heals with neoadjuvant treatment (*see* Fig. 7.9).
- Metaphyseal tumours in contact with part of the growth plate. Intra-epiphyseal osteotomy could be an alternative to the "three-step variant" of the technique (*see* Chap. 8).
- Metaphyseal tumours without involvement of the physis, but in patients who are close to the end of growth. In such patients, it is more difficult to achieve physeal distraction.

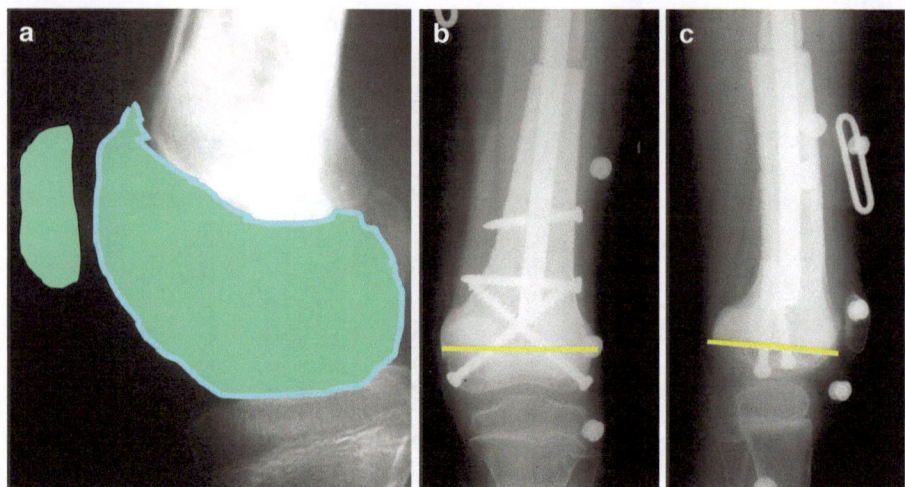

Fig. 10.6 (**a**) The growth plate extends to the cartilage of the condyles and *trochlea femoralis*. (**b**, **c**) Patient came to our hospital after pulmonary metastases had been detected by another institution. Previous X-ray was not available to us. Apparently, intra-epiphyseal osteotomy had been performed to preserve the joint. The functional result was poor because the osteotomy line cut the *trochlea*

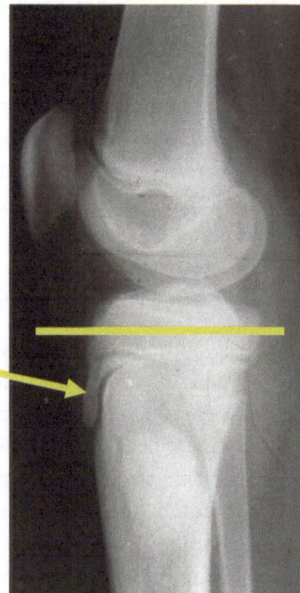

Proximal tibia:
Patellar tendon
atachment

Fig. 10.7 Intra-epiphyseal osteotomy does not allow preservation of the patellar tendon attachment

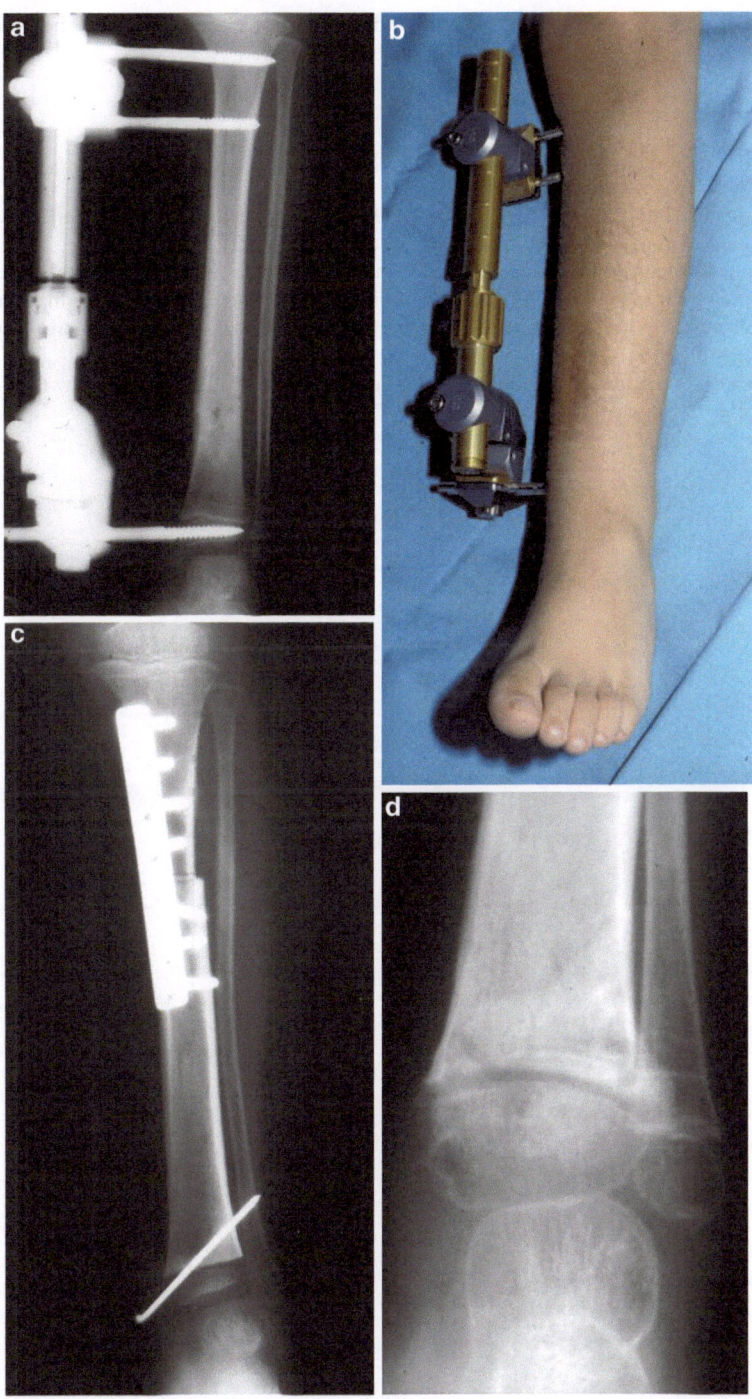

Fig. 10.8 (**a, b**) Physeal distraction before excision of a Ewing's sarcoma in the distal tibia of a 3-year-old boy (the youngest patient in the series). (**c, d**) The growth plate remains active after removal of the distal Kirschner wire

10

Some examples relating to the second and the third of these criteria are shown in Figs. 10.1 and 10.2.

References

1. Manfrini M. Intraepiphyseal resection. In: Albiñana J, ed. Bone Tumors in Children and Adolescents. *Rev Mapfre Medicina*. 1997;8(Suppl. I)282–283.
2. Capanna R, Manfrini M, Ceruso M, et al. A new reconstruction for metaphyseal resections: a combined graft (allograft shell plus vascularized fibula). Preliminary results. In: Brown, ed. Complications in Limb Salvage. Prevention, Management and Outcome. Montreal: Publisher ISOLS; 1991:319.
3. De Pablos J, Cañadell J. Experimental physeal distraction in immature sheep. *Clin Orthop*. 1990;250:73–80.

Questions and Answers

11

Mikel San-Julian

Abstract The technique of physeal distraction before tumour excision has been described at several national and international meetings, where it has invariably aroused considerable interest. This chapter deals with some of the questions put forward at these meetings.

- **Does this technique mean any delay in the protocol for treatment of the tumour?**
  Answer: No.

  You can place the external fixator during the course of pre-operative chemotherapy. You need only 15 min to place the external fixator, 15 days before the established date for surgery. The external fixator allows the patient to continue with his or her normal life, and of course, it does not impede adherence to chemotherapy protocols, even intra-arterial procedures.

- **Do you employ the technique in all cases of metaphyseal bone tumours?**
  From: Antonie Tamineau, University of Leyden, The Netherlands
  In: SICOT, 1996 Meeting, Amsterdam
  Answer: No.

  It is a technique for selected cases: those cases of metaphyseal bone tumours in which the tumour has not crossed the growth plate. If the tumour has crossed the growth plate, the joint should be dealt with reconstructive surgery (arthrodesis, prosthesis, or osteoarticular allograft).

- **What is the reason for the distraction technique?**
  From: Zdenek Matejowsky Sr., Praga
  In: EMSOS, 1994 Meeting, Amsterdam
  Answer: The anatomy of the growth plate.

  The growth plate seems to represent a temporary barrier to tumour spread. The growth plate is not a plane surface and so it is difficult to be sure that an intra-epiphyseal osteotomy has not passed through the tumour and left tumoural tissue behind.

Mikel San-Julian
Department of Orthopedic Surgery, University Clinic of Navarra, Avda. Pio XII, s/n, Pamplona, Navarra 31008, Spain
e-mail: msjulian@unav.es

J. Cañadell and M. San-Julian (eds.), *Pediatric Bone Sarcomas: Epiphysiolysis Before Excision*,   **145**
DOI: 10.1007/978-1-84882-130-9_11, © Springer-Verlag London Limited 2011

- **What about the risk of infection?**

From: Mario Campanacci, Bologna

In: ISOLS, 1995 Meeting, Firenze

  Answer: The risk is the same as with other reconstructive surgery.

  The risk of infection is no higher in tumour pathology than that in other reconstructive surgery. Obviously, patients are immunosuppressed as a result of the chemotherapy, but the external fixator is only used for 10–15 days. Not even in cases where we used an external fixator as a support for autografting or bone transport (see Chap. 9), have we had any related problems with infection. Seven percent of patients suffered an infection of the reconstruction during the follow-up; this rate is no higher than that in our own overall series of allografts or prosthesis, or that reported by other authors.

- **Could you exploit the procedure to achieve some lengthening before resection?**

From: Marco Manfrini, Bologna

In: EMSOS, 1997 Meeting, Münster

  Answer: No.

  The technique is just an epiphysiolysis in order to achieve a good margin for resection of the tumour. It is not a lengthening procedure. The tumour should be resected as soon as possible. Other techniques exist for avoiding or correcting limb-length discrepancies after tumour resection.

- **Could this technique stimulate tumour growth?**

From: Wilfred Winkelman, Münster

In: EMSOS, 1997 Meeting, Münster

  Answer: No.

  The disruption of the growth plate occurs suddenly after several days of distraction. We do not believe that this stimulates tumour growth.

- **Does chemotherapy influence callus formation?**

From: Wilfred Winkelman, University of Münster

In: EMSOS, 1997 Meeting, Münster

  Answer: What callus?

  The technique is simply epiphysiolysis in order to achieve a good resection margin; there is no need to wait for callus formation.

  Chemotherapy, of course, plays an important role in the consolidation of allografts and the callus formation in bone transport procedures (see Chap. 9), but the epiphysiolysis before resection of the tumour is not a procedure concerned with callus formation.

- **Are there any age limits for the procedure?**

From: Name unknown

In: EMSOS, 1997 Meeting, Münster

  Answer: Appropriacy has to be determined on a patient by patient basis.

  The youngest patient in which the technique has been used was 3 years old (see Fig. 10.8), but malignant bone tumours are not frequently seen in children so young. The oldest patient in the series was 15 years old. Before applying the technique, one has to ascertain that the growth plate is still active and that the patient has not finished growing.

- **Has the technique been employed in litic lesions?**

From: Becker, Münster

In: EMSOS, 1997 Meeting, Münster

Answer: Yes.

Osteogenic sarcoma and Ewing's sarcoma, the two bone tumours most frequently seen in childhood, are not usually litic lesions. However, we have successfully used the technique with litic lesions such as telangiectatic osteosarcoma (see Fig. 9.11). In such cases, it is important to be sure that there is no pathological fracture.

- **Has the technique been employed in metaphyseal tumours which were seen to be in contact with the growth plate in the MRI scans?**

From: Name unknown

In: SICOT, 1996 Meeting, Amsterdam

Answer: Yes.

The most important thing is to be sure that the tumour has not crossed the growth plate. In cases of contact between the tumour and the physis, you can also use the "three steps" technique.

- **Does the retained growth plate remain active after the distraction procedure?**

From: Marco Manfrini, Bologna

In: EMSOS, 1997 Meeting, Münster

Answer: In some cases.

As reported by De Pablos et al. from our department, if physeal distraction is used as a lengthening procedure, the growth plate may continue growing when lengthening is performed at a rate of 1–1.5 mm/day. In cases of epiphysiolysis for preserving the epiphysis, it is also possible that the growth plate will continue growing; Chap. 9 presents some cases that demonstrate subsequent growth. However, arrest of growth could be caused by other factors such as radiotherapy, delayed weight bearing, and the osteosynthesis device used for stabilisation of the retained epiphysis (see Chap. 9).

- **Osteosynthesis of the allograft with a locked nail will not allow subsequent growth!**

From: Rodolfo Capanna, Firenze

In: ISOLS, 1996 Meeting, Firenze

Answer: True.

We used this kind of osteosynthesis device in patients who were nearing the end of growth. Allografts which were 1.5–2 cm longer than the resected piece were employed in an attempt to minimize the final limb-length discrepancy. We preferred this approach to osteosynthesis for the older patients in our series because it eliminates the risk of allograft fracture. However, in young children, we prefer minimal osteosynthesis devices of the epiphysis, such as Kirschner wires or the distal end of two Enders, to permit later growth (see Chap. 9).

- **How could you be sure about tumour extension before the MRI era?**

From: William Enneking, University of Gainesville (Florida)

In: ISOLS, 1995 Meeting, Firenze

Answer: Sometimes we could not be sure, so we used a modified surgical procedure.

Before the advent of MRI, we used the other imaging methods, such as CT, scintigraphy, X-ray, and angiography when otherwise needed. In cases where we found ourselves left in any doubt about whether the tumour was compromising the physis, we employed a variant of the technique with three surgical steps that enabled us to accommodate a histological inspection of the distracted margin (see Chap. 8). Nowadays, we believe that, owing to the accuracy of MRI, this is not necessary in most cases.

- **I believe that there is usually a high risk of local recurrence; how many of your patients had a follow-up longer than 2 years?**

From: William Enneking, University of Gainesville (Florida)

In: ISOLS, 1995 Meeting, Firenze

   Answer: Most of them.

When Dr. Enneking put this question to us, he suggested that we had been lucky to have had no local recurrences. We have been employing the technique since 1984, and so the first patient in the series has now 24 years of follow-up. The technique has been used in almost more than 130 patients and we have had no cases of local recurrence in the retained epiphysis.

- **What happens if the distraction does not take place correctly?**

From: Ulrich Exner, Zurich (Switzerland)

   Answer: Intra-epiphyseal osteotomy can still be performed.

Although distraction is possible even in litic tumours, in a couple of cases pathological fracture has occurred during distraction. In these cases, we carried out an intra-epiphyseal osteotomy to remove the tumour. There were no complications, no local recurrence, and function was good.

- **Given the proven safety and the excellent results, why is this technique not more widely adopted?**

From: Name unknown.

In: ISOLS, 2007 Meeting, Hamburg

   Answer: Confidence in the technique requires very different types of specialist knowledge and experience.

I think there are two main reasons why the technique has not been more widely adopted. First, orthopaedic oncologists are not necessarily accustomed to dealing with techniques such as external fixation, growth plate surgery, and lengthening procedures, because such surgeons concentrate primarily on tumour surgery. Without a clear understanding of how the growth plate breaks when distraction is slowly applied, a surgeon focussed on resection may find it difficult to muster sufficient trust that epiphysiolysis can provide a safe margin of resection in bone sarcomas. Cañadell had a wide experience in paediatric orthopaedics, external fixation, and many other fields of orthopaedics, and it was perhaps this broad familiarity which enabled him to conceive of and develop his technique. Second, in many centres, the indications for amputation have only diminished very slowly during the last two decades; to stop amputating bone tumours requires considerable confidence in the efficiency of chemotherapy. Professor Cañadell was exceptional in his decision to stop amputating bone tumours once he knew of this efficiency. When he started this technique for preserving the joint, most people simply did not believe it was possible without diminishing the chances of survival.

Nowadays, although not globally accepted, the technique is being used in many cancer centres around the world including centres in Seville, Barcelona, Madrid and Valencia (Spain), Zurich (Switzerland), Leiden (the Netherlands), Tokyo (Japan), Gothenburg (Sweden), Pernanbuco (Brazil), Bologna (Italy), etc.

Index